MEDICAL
SPANISH

MEDICAL SPANISH

Second Edition

GAIL L. BONGIOVANNI, M.D.
The Jewish Hospital of Cincinnati
The Christ Hospital of Cincinnati

Revised with the assistance of
Ariel Dan Teitel, M.D.
Hospital for Special Surgery
New York, New York

McGRAW-HILL, INC.
Health Professions Division
New York St. Louis San Francisco Auckland Bogotá
Caracas Lisbon London Madrid Mexico Milan
Montreal New Delhi Paris San Juan Singapore
Sydney Tokyo Toronto

MEDICAL SPANISH

8 9 0 DOC DOC 9 8 7 6

This book was set in Souvenir by Precision Graphics, Inc. The editors
were J. Dereck Jeffers and Lester A. Sheinis. The production supervisor
was Richard Ruzycka. The cover was designed by N.S.G. Design.
R. R. Donnelley & Sons Company was printer and binder.

ISBN 0-07-006489-X

Library of Congress Cataloging-in-Publication Data

Bongiovanni, Gail.
   Medical Spanish / Gail L. Bongiovanni, revised with the assistance
of Ariel Dan Teitel.—2d ed.
      p. cm.
   Includes indexes.
   ISBN 0-07-006489-X
   1. Spanish language—Conversation and phrase books (for medical
personnel) 2. Medical—Terminology. I. Teitel, Ariel Dan.
II. Title.
   [DNLM: 1. Medicine—phrases—Spanish. W 15 B713m]
PC4120.M3B6   1991
468.2'421—dc20
DNLM/DLC
for Library of Congress   91–15613
                                                             CIP

To My Parents . . . because of the
love and respect we share.

Contents

Preface

Medical Spanish was written to express my gratitude to those people of Spain and Latin America who, since 1967, have given me the opportunity to share their language and their spirit of life.

Since its first publication in 1978, *Medical Spanish* has assisted English-speaking medical personnel as they tried to communicate and administer health care to their Spanish-speaking patients.

This second edition of *Medical Spanish* continues the comprehensive yet simple linguistic approach that allows medical personnel to take a thorough medical history and perform a complete medical examination on their Spanish-speaking patients. The book has been revised to include questions on drug abuse, AIDS, and other sexually transmitted diseases.

My special thanks go to Dr. Ariel Dan Teitel for his assistance in revising *Medical Spanish*.

MEDICAL
SPANISH

Chapter 1
HOW TO USE
THIS BOOK

Medical Spanish, formerly entitled *Entre Doctor y Paciente*,[1] was written to aid English-speaking medical personnel working with Spanish-speaking patients. This book is intended to provide a practical method for improving communication.

This book was prepared in Guatemala City, Guatemala. Practical trials were carried out for two months at Roosevelt Hospital, Guatemala City, where effectiveness of the text was tested in patient interviews.

[1] *Between Doctor and Patient.*

1

1.1 ENGLISH INTO SPANISH

The vocabulary presented is representative of Spanish as it is spoken in Spain and Latin America. The English phrases have not always been given a literal translation. Instead, the Spanish words and phrases have been chosen to communicate the sense of the English questions in a way that will be understood by the patient.

Example:

I am going to examine your . . .

Voy a examinarle su . . .

1 abdomen*.

1 *estómago* (stomach).

Here the English word "abdomen" is translated as "estómago" (stomach). Wherever such free translating is done, the words involved are marked by an asterisk, and the literal translation of the Spanish word is given in parentheses. In this way, the interviewer will not read one word in English and think the same word has been translated literally into Spanish.

In order to keep the English and the Spanish phrases structurally similar, it was necessary, in some instances, to use a slightly awkward English wording. The Spanish phrase, however, is worded correctly and naturally.

Example:

Is the diarrhea . . .

La *diarrea es* . . .

1 of what color?
2 with blood?
3 with fat?

1 de qué *color*?
2 con *sangre*?
3 con *grasa*?

Thus, if interviewers follow the Spanish translation presented in the text, they will be speaking grammatically and idiomatically.

1.2 ORGANIZATION OF THE BOOK

The text is divided into twelve chapters. Several chapters have been subdivided into sections to facilitate the collection of information. For the chapters on review of systems and physical examination, each section is devoted to one organ system. Certain sections have been further subdivided.

Example:
Chapter 5 Chief Complaint or Review of Systems
Section 5.4 Gastrointestinal System
Section 5.4.1 Nutritional History

Chapter 2 introduces some essentials of Spanish grammar. The Appendix presents basic and supplemental vocabulary.

The remainder of the text is to be used during an interview with a patient who comes to the clinic or hospital. The interview begins with questions about the patient's social and family history (Chapter 3). Questions on past medical history, review of systems, physical examination, general treatment and follow-up, and medical therapy are covered in Chapters 4 to 8. Three special chapters cover the topics of contraception, labor and delivery, and poisonings.

1.3 THE INTERVIEW FORMAT

For the interviewer with little knowledge of Spanish, a response to an open-ended question may be difficult to understand. To avoid confusion, the questions to the patient have been phrased so that they can be answered either "Yes" ("Sí") or "No" ("No"). Several variations on the yes/no question are also used. To round out the interview, a multipurpose request format, which is to be accompanied by appropriate gestures, is provided.

1.3.1 Basic Yes/No Question

Almost all questions in this book are phrased so that the patient may answer "Sí" or "No" as the interviewer reads them. Some questions begin with a repeating phrase to which a list of different words or phrases may be appended.

Example:

Do you often . . .	Tiene *frecuentemente*
1 feel nauseated?	1 náusea
2 vomit?	2 *vómitos?*
3 burp?	3 *eructos?*

The interviewer is not supposed to *suggest* symptoms to the patient. He simply asks, "Do you often feel *nauseated?*" and *waits* for the patient to respond "Sí" or "No." Other questions give more detailed information, but the basic format is the same.

Example:

Do you have pain on urination . . .	Tiene *dolor* al orinar . . .
1 at the beginning?	1 al *empezar?*
2 the whole time?	2 *todo* el tiempo?
3 at the end?	3 al *terminar?*

This method may alter the usual dialogue between health worker and patient, but it also helps the interviewer obtain information. If the traditional "open-ended" question form is used, it is difficult to restrain the patient from speaking too rapidly, and the interviewer with a limited acquaintance with Spanish will be unable to understand the response.

Three variations of the yes/no question are also employed.

1.3.2 Double-Tense Question

This question format is very practical for someone just learning Spanish. By substituting verb tenses, the interviewer can use the "double-tense questions" to obtain twice as much information. With this method of questioning either the *chief complaint or review of systems* (Chapter 5) can be investigated. The interviewer uses the same questions, but changes the tense.

Example:

Do you have OR have you had . . .	*Tiene* O *ha tenido* . . .
1 pain in your chest?	1 dolor del pecho?
2 shortness of breath?	2 sensación de ahogo?
3 difficulty in breathing?	3 dificultad al respirar?
4 night sweats?	4 sudor por la noche?

This techinque is easy to use and does not require the interviewer to learn a completely new vocabulary. In a very few instances, a question is illogical in one tense. The interviewer should be alert to this possibility and carefully select the tense to be used. The interviewer should *not* ask "Do you have or have you had. . . ." If the chief complaint is under investigation, the interviewer asks, "Do you have. . . ." If the review of systems is being covered, the interviewer chooses "Have you had. . . ."

1.3.3 One-Common-Phrase Question

Another variation of the basic yes/no question format is the one-common-phrase question. In this variation, the same introductory phrase is used with different words to elicit additional information.

Example:

Have you ever been hit in the . . .

Se ha *golpeado* en . . .

1 head?	1 la cabeza?
2 face?	2 la cara?
3 neck?	3 el cuello?
4 eyes?	4 los ojos?

This question format may change the usual dialogue between health worker and patient but, again, it does simplify and perhaps eliminate the difficulty an English-speaking person may experience in interpreting a Spanish answer.

1.3.4 Fill-In-the-Blank Question

This question format is a version of the one-common-phrase approach. On the basis of responses made previously by the patient, the interviewer can gain additional information simply by substituting the known information into the question.

Example:

In reviewing the cardiovascular system, the interviewer has learned that the patient has experienced "shortness of breath." To obtain additional information about this symptom, the blank in the question is filled in with the known symptom.

Was (Is) the *shortness of breath* accompanied by . . .	Se acompañó (acompaña) *la sensación de ahogo* con . . .
1 fever?	1 *fiebre?*
2 trembling?	2 *temblores?*
3 sweating?	3 *sudores?*

In this example, the combined used of the double-tense question and the fill-in-the-blank question provides the interviewer with more extensive information on the patient's problem.

1.3.5 The Multipurpose Request

The request format allows the examiner to communicate several different instructions with the same phrase. This type of presentation is particularly helpful during the physical examination. When using these questions, the interviewer must *actively point to or demonstrate* a particular item.

Example:

Please . . .	Por favor . . .
1 walk on THIS.	1 camine en ESTO.

This refers to a treadmill for the exercise tolerance test.

2 take THESE pills.	2 tome ESTAS pildoras.

These refers to a specific color or shape of the pills.

Whenever the multipurpose request is used in the book, the variable is shown in capitals as in the examples shown here.

The yes/no question, together with its variations, and the multipurpose request are employed to facilitate the interview, physical examination, and follow-up. This method of interviewing is simple and requires only that the interviewer be a more active participant in the clinic or a hospital visit. For those health workers with a greater knowledge of Spanish, the book provides an ample medical vocabulary, and it should not be difficult for such workers to incorporate the new vocabulary into their usual interview.

Effective communication in a linguistically simple style is the principal goal of this book. The interview format has been designed to minimize the interviewer's difficulty as he or she attempts to communicate in a new language with patients. The primary aim of *Medical Spanish* is to help the English-speaking health worker provide more reassuring and effective health care to Spanish-speaking patients.

Chapter 2
GRAMMAR AND PRONUNCIATION

This book is not intended to provide complete grammatical information. Therefore, there are only a few concepts to keep in mind about grammar and pronunciation.

The syllabic breakdown of the Spanish words is not given. It is recommended that the words be pronounced as they would be in English, keeping the few pronunciation rules in mind. Emphasis is indicated in key Spanish words or phrases by an underscore. The patient will understand even though the accent may not be perfect.

2.1 PRONUNCIATION

1 Spanish vowels:
   a   is pronounced like "a" in *fAther.*
   e   is pronounced like "ey" in *thEY.*
   i   is pronounced like "ee" in *frEE.*
   o   is pronounced like "o" in *lOw.*
   u   is pronounced like "oe" in *shOE.*

2 When "a," "e," or "o" is followed by "u" or "i," the two vowels form a single sound with prolongation of the "a," "e," or "o" sound.

Example: c<u>a</u>usa (cause)[1]

When "i" or "u" precedes another vowel, the two vowels form one sound with slight emphasis of the second vowel.

Example: vi<u>u</u>da (widow)

3 "B" and "v" are pronounced exactly alike in Spanish. They sound like the "b" in *a*B*olition*.

4 "Ch" is an independent letter of the alphabet and is pronounced like the hard "ch" in *CHeese*.

5 At the beginning of a word, "d" is like the hard "d" in *day*. In the middle of a word, "d" is pronounced like the "th" in *wiTH*.

Example: Todo (all) is pronounced "<u>toe</u>-tho."

6 In Spanish the "h" is *always* silent.

Example: Hijo (son) is pronounced "<u>ee</u>-ho." All other letters are pronounced.

7 "J" is similar to the hard "h" in *horizon* and is slightly guttural.

Example: Joven (young) is pronounced "<u>ho</u>-ven."

8 A "ll" is a separate letter of the alphabet and is pronounced like "ye" in *YEllow*.

Example: Llamar (call) is pronounced "<u>ya</u>-mar."

9 "Ñ" is a separate letter of the alphabet. It is pronounced like "ny" of *caNYon* and is nasal-sounding.

10 Single "r" at the beginning of a word and "rr" in the middle of a word are always trilled. This sound is made by vibrating the tongue against the roof of the mouth with a strong expulsion of breath.

---

[1]The English translation is always enclosed in parentheses. Underlinings of the Spanish words indicate where the *accent* will fall.

11 If a word ends in a consonant other than "n" or "s," the stress is on the last syllable.

Example: ard<u>or</u> (burning)

Words ending in a vowel, "n," or "s" stress the second to the last syllable.

Example: ca<u>m</u>isa (shirt), <u>ca</u>sas (houses)

Any word whose pronunciation differs from these rules will always have a *written accent.*

Example: médico (doctor), not me<u>di</u>co.

2.2 GRAMMAR

1 Plurals of nouns are formed simply by adding "s" if the word ends in an unaccented vowel.

Example: <u>de</u>do (finger)
    <u>de</u>dos (fingers)

or by adding "es" if it ends in a consonant, "y," or an accented vowel.

Example: dol<u>or</u> (pain)
    dol<u>or</u>es (pains)
    ley (law)
    <u>le</u>yes (laws)
    rubí (ruby)
    rubíes (rubies)

2 The definite articles are:

Feminine		**Masculine**	
Singular	Plural	Singular	Plural
la	las	el	los

Example: la <u>pier</u>na (the leg)
    las <u>pier</u>nas (the legs)
    el <u>bra</u>zo (the arm)
    los <u>bra</u>zos (the arms)

3 In general, words ending in "o" are masculine and those ending in "a" are feminine. An adjective agrees in number and in gender with the noun it modifies.

>*Example:* <u>ni</u>ña *(girl)*   las <u>ni</u>ñas enfermas (the sick girls)
>
>   <u>ni</u>ño *(boy)*   el <u>ni</u>ño enfermo (the sick boy)

One relevant exception to this rule is: la <u>ma</u>no (the hand) rather than el mano.

4 *Possessive Adjectives:* Unless you are speaking to a child, you should use the formal address.

	Singular	*Plural*
(my)	mi	mis
(your familiar)	tu	tus
(his, her, your formal)	su	sus
(our)	<u>nue</u>stro (a)[2]	<u>neu</u>stros (as)[3]
(your familiar)	<u>vue</u>stro (a)	<u>vue</u>stros (as)
(their)	su	sus

For parts of the body the possessive adjective can be replaced by the definite article. The meaning of the sentence remains clear.

>*Example:* Le<u>van</u>te su <u>bra</u>zo. (Raise your arm.)
>
>   *or*
>
>   Le<u>van</u>te el <u>bra</u>zo. (still understood as, Raise your arm.)

5 *Subject Pronouns*

	Singular		*Plural*
(I)	yo	(we)	no<u>so</u>tros (as)
(you familiar)	tú	(you familiar)	vo<u>so</u>tros (as)
(he)	él[4]	(they)	<u>e</u>llos (as)
(she)	<u>e</u>lla		
(you formal)	us<u>ted</u>[5]	(you formal)	us<u>te</u>des

[2]The feminine form is made by changing the final "o" to an "a."
[3]The plural is formed by adding "s."
[4]Notice the written accent on él (he) to distinguish it from el (the).
[5]Usted is abbreviated Vd., ustedes is abbreviated Vds.

It is not always necessary to write the subject pronoun in a sentence. The conjugated verb is enough.

Example: Yo soy el médico. (I am the doctor.) can correctly be written, Soy el médico.

6   *Contractions*

al = a + el (to the)
del = de + el (of the) It also forms the possessive.

Example: Voy al hospital. (I am going to the hospital.)
la herida del paciente (the patient's wound)
(the wound *of the* patient)

7   *Common Suffixes and Prefixes*

a   *Diminutives:* "ito" (a) dolor (pain)
dolorcito (slight pain)

b   *Augmentatives:* "ísimo" (a) cansado (tired)
cansadísimo (very tired)

c   *Adverbs:* "mente" is added to the feminine form of the adjective to form the adverb.

generosa (generous)
generosamente (generously)

d   *"Dad" and "tad"* are equivalent to the English "ty."

cantidad (quantity)
facultad (faculty)

e   *"Ería"* denotes the location where something is made or sold.

libro (book)
librería (bookstore)

f   *"Ero"* (a) indicates the person who makes or sells the object.

zapato (shoe)
zapatero (shoemaker)

g   *"Des"* before a word forms the opposite of the original word.

vest<u>ir</u> (to dress)
desvest<u>ir</u> (to undress)
agra<u>d</u>able (agreeable)
desagra<u>d</u>able (disagreeable)

2.3 SPELLING

To spell any word in Spanish, write it exactly as it sounds, remembering that the "h" is silent. Normally, only three letters may be doubled in Spanish:

c   contracción (contraction)
l   <u>ell</u>a (she)
r   h<u>ierr</u>o (iron)

Chapter 3
SOCIAL AND
FAMILY HISTORY

3.1   GENERAL SOCIAL BACKGROUND

What is your name?
How old are you?
Where were you born?
When did you come to this country?
Where do you live?
How long have you lived there?
What is your address?
Have you lived in _____?
Do you live alone?

DATOS SOCIALES GENERALES

Cómo se llama usted?[1]
Cuántos años tiene?
Donde nació?
Cuándo vino usted a este país?
Dónde vive?
Hace *cuánto* tiempo que vive allí?
Cuál es su dirección?
Vivió usted en _____?
Vive *solo* (a)?

[1]For the sake of simplicity, the inverted question mark, which should *precede* every question, has been omitted.

Do you live with your . . .

1 parents?
2 husband (wife)?
3 son (daughter)?
4 mother?
5 father?
6 uncle (aunt)?
7 grandfather
  (grandmother)?
8 cousin?
9 friend?
10 other relative?

Are you . . .

1 single?
2 married?
3 separated?
4 divorced?
5 widowed?
6 single, but living with
  your girlfriend
  (boyfriend)?

Do you consider yourself to
be

1 homosexual?
2 bisexual?
3 heterosexual?

Do you have any children?
How many?
What ages?
Have you ever been married
before?
How many different partners
do you have in a month?
Do you have anal intercourse?

Vive con . . .

1 sus padres?
2 su esposo (a)?
3 su hijo (a)?
4 su madre?
5 su padre?
6 su tío (a)?
7 su abuelo (a)?

8 un (a) primo (a)?
9 un (a) amigo (a)?
10 otro pariente?

Es . . .

1 soltero (a)?
2 casado (a)?
3 separado (a)?
4 divorciado (a)?
5 viudo (a)?
6 soltero (a), pero vive con
  su novia (o)?

Se considera

1 homosexual?
2 bisexual?
3 heterosexual?

Tiene *hijos*?
Cuántos?
De qué *edades*?
Ha estado casado (a) *alguna
vez*?
Cuántos amantes tiene por
mes?
Practica coito anal?

Do you have . . .	Tiene . . .
1 primary education?	1 una educación *primaria*?
2 secondary education?	2 una educación *secundaria*?
3 college education?	3 una educación *universitaria*?
4 graduate education?	4 una educación *graduada*?
5 professional education?	5 una educación *profesional*?
6 occupational education?	6 una educación *especializada*?

Is your religion . . .	Su religión es . . .
1 Catholic?	1 Católica?
2 Protestant?	2 Protestante?
3 Jewish?	3 Judía?
4 Baptist?	4 Bautista?
5 Mormon?	5 Mormón?
6 Evangelist?	6 Evangélica?
7 Episcopalian?	7 Episcopal?
8 Christian Science?	8 Ciencia Cristiana?
9 Jehovah's Witness?	9 Testigo de Jehová?
10 Muslim?	10 Musulmán?
11 Buddhist?	11 Budísta?
12 Hindu?	12 Hindú?

3.2 OCCUPATIONAL HISTORY

DATOS OCUPACIONALES

Do you work outside your home?
What type of work do (did) you do?

Trabaja afuera de su casa?

En *qué* trabaja (trabajaba)?

1 retired	1 jubilado (a)
2 teacher	2 maestro (a)
3 secretary	3 secretaria

4	housewife	4	ama de casa	
5	salesperson	5	vendedor (a)	
6	doctor	6	médico, doctor (a)	
7	lawyer	7	abogado	
8	engineer	8	ingeniero (a)	
9	student	9	estudiante	
10	architect	10	arquitecto (a)	
11	accountant	11	contador (a)	
12	farmer	12	campesino, agricultor	
13	waiter (waitress)	13	camarero (a)	
14	mechanic	14	mecánico (a)	
15	factory worker	15	trabajador (a) de fábrica	
16	truck driver	16	conductor (a) de camión	
17	bus driver	17	conductor (a) de bus	
18	taxi driver	18	conductor (a) de taxi	

Where do (did) you work?

En *dónde* trabaja (trabajaba)?

How long have you worked there?

Hace *cuánto* tiempo que trabaja allí?

What was your first job?

Cuál fue su *primer* empleo?

What other jobs have you had?

Qué *otros* empleos ha tenido?

How long did you work there?

Cuánto tiempo trabajó en eso?

Why did you change jobs?

Por qué cambió de trabajo?

Are you happy in your work? Why?

Está *contento* (a) en su trabajo? Por qué?

Do (Did) you work with . . .

En su trabajo, está (estaba) *en contacto con* . . .

1	lead?	1	plomo?
2	insecticides?	2	insecticidas?
3	chemicals?	3	substancias *químicas*?
4	paints?	4	pinturas?
5	plastics?	5	plasticos?

6	other synthetic materials?		6	otras substancias *sintéticas?*
7	drugs?		7	drogas?
8	dusts?		8	polvos?
9	animals?		9	animales?
10	birds		10	pájaros?
11	radiation?		11	irradiación?

When?
For how long?
Do (Did) you use any precautionary measures?
What?

Cuándo?
Por cuánto tiempo?
Toma (tomaba) *precauciones?*
Cuáles?

3.3 HOBBIES AND SOCIAL ORGANIZATIONS

Do you enjoy . . .

1 sports?
2 reading?
3 movies?
4 music?
5 theater?
6 painting?
7 photography?

Do you play an instrument?

Do you belong to groups of . . .

1 the church?
2 the school?
3 sports?

PASATIEMPOS Y ORGANIZACIONES SOCIALES

Le gusta . . .

1 el deporte?
2 leer?
3 el cine?
4 la música?
5 el teatro?
6 la pintura?
7 la fotografía?

Toca un instrumento?

Pertenece a grupos de . . .

1 la iglesia?
2 la escuela?
3 deportes?

3.4 INSURANCE AND ECONOMIC INFORMATION

Are you the sole financial support of your family?
About how much money do you earn a month?
Does anyone else in the family work?
Who?
How much do they earn?

Do you receive financial assistance from any . . .

1 other people?
2 organizations?

Do you have . . .

1 life insurance?
2 hospital insurance?
3 accident insurance?
4 Medicare?
5 Blue Shield?
6 Blue Cross?

SEGUROS E INFORMACIÓN ECONÓMICA

Es el *único* que sostiene a su familia?
Más o menos, *cuánto* gana mensualmente?
Hay alquién *más* en la familia que trabaja?
Quién?
Cuánto ganan ellos?

Recibe *ayuda financiera* de . . .

1 alguna *otra* persona?
2 alguna *organización?*

Tiene *seguros* . . .

1 de vida?
2 para el hospital?
3 para accidentes?
4 de Medicare?
5 de Blue Shield?
6 de Blue Cross?

Chapter 4
PAST MEDICAL HISTORY

This chapter covers the traditional information needed for a complete medical background. There are questions on immunizations, foreign travel, and illnesses that may have been acquired abroad.

4.1 PAST HEALTH, HOSPITALIZATIONS, AND ILLNESSES

How has your health been up until now . . .

1 good?
2 fair?
3 poor?

ESTADO DE SALUD, HOSPITALIZACIONES Y ENFERMEDADES ANTERIORES

Hasta *ahora*, cómo ha estado su salud . . .

1 buena?
2 regular?
3 mala?

Do you have your own
doctor?

Tiene su *propio* médico?

What is his (her) . . .

Cuál es su . . .

1 name?
2 address?
3 telephone number?

1 no<u>m</u>bre?
2 dire<u>cció</u>n?
3 *nú*mero de tel<u>é</u>fono?

When was the last time you
went to his (her) office?

Cuándo fue la <u>úl</u>tima vez
que fue a su clínica?

What was the visit for?

Por qué consultó a su
médico?

Have you ever been in the
hospital?

Ha estado en el *hosp<u>it</u>al*?

When was it?

Cu<u>án</u>do?

Why were you there?

Por qué?

How long were you there?

Cuánto tiempo estuvo allí?

Which hospital was it?

En qué hospital?

What is the address?

Cuál es la *dire<u>cción</u>?*

Have you ever had surgery?

Ha sido *oper<u>a</u>do* (a) alguna
vez?

Did they operate . . .

Le *oper<u>a</u>ron* de . . .

1 on your tonsils?
2 on your appendix?
3 on your gallbladder?
4 on your uterus?
5 on your prostate?
6 for cataracts?
7 on your ovaries . . .
   a the right one?
   b the left one?
   c both?
8 for a hernia . . .
   a inguinal?
   b femoral?

1 las amí<u>g</u>dalas?
2 el ap<u>é</u>ndice?
3 la ves<u>í</u>cula bil<u>iar</u>?
4 la ma<u>triz</u>?
5 la pr<u>ós</u>tata?
6 cata<u>ra</u>tas?
7 los o<u>v</u>arios . . .
   a el de<u>re</u>cho?
   b el izquierdo?
   c <u>am</u>bos?
8 una <u>her</u>nia . . .
   a ingui<u>nal</u>?
   b femo<u>ral</u>?

9 on your kidneys . . .
   a for stones?
   b for removal?
   c for transplant?

Have you had . . .

1 chicken pox?
2 measles?
3 rubella?[1]
4 mumps?
5 whooping cough?
6 scarlet fever?
7 rheumatic fever?
8 tuberculosis?
9 hepatitis?

4.2 IMMUNIZATIONS AND ILLNESSES ABROAD

Have you ever traveled outside this country?
When?
Where?
Were you sick?
Did you see a doctor?

What was . . .

1 the diagnosis?
2 the treatment?

Have you had vaccinations for . . .

  1 diphtheria?
  2 whooping cough?

9 los riñones . . .
   a por cálculos?
   b le quitaron?
   c para transplante?

Ha tenido . . .

1 varicela?
2 sarampión?
3 rubeola?[1]
4 paperas?
5 tos ferina?
6 escarlatina?
7 fiebre reumática?
8 tuberculosis?
9 hepatitis?

INMUNIZACIONES Y ENFERMEDADES AL EXTRANJERO

Ha viajado *fuera* de este país?
Cuándo?
A dónde?
Se enfermó?
Le vió un médico?

Cuál fue . . .

1 el diagnóstico?
2 el tratamiento?

Le han puesto vacunas de . . .

  1 difteria?
  2 tos ferina?

---

[1]The translation of rubella into Spanish is rubeola. This is not a copy error.

3	polio?		3	polio?
4	tetanus?		4	tétano?
5	smallpox?		5	viruela?
6	typhoid fever?		6	fiebre tifoidea?
7	cholera?		7	cólera?
8	BCG?		8	BCG?
9	yellow fever?		9	fiebre amarilla?
10	rubella?		10	rubeola?
11	measles?		11	sarampión?

When were they?
When was your chest x-ray?

Where was it taken?

Were the results . . .

1 normal?
2 abnormal?

Have you been tested for tuberculosis?
When?
Who tested you?

Were the results . . .

1 positive?
2 negative?

Have you had a blood transfusion?

Cuándo?
Cuándo le tomaron su última *radiografía* del tórax?
Dónde se la sacaron?

Los *resultados* fueron . . .

1 normales?
2 anormales?

Ha recibido la prueba de *tuberculina*?
Cuándo?
Quién le dio la prueba?

Los resultados fueron . . .

1 positivos?
2 negativos?

Ha recibido alguna transfusión de sangre?

4.3 SOCIAL HABITS

Do you ever have problems sleeping?
How is your appetite?

Do you smoke/Have you ever smoked . . .

HÁBITOS SOCIALES

Duerme *bien*?

Cómo está su *apetito*?

Fuma/Alguna vez fumó . . .

1 cigarettes?
2 pipe?
3 cigars?
4 marijuana?

How much do you smoke a day?

How long have you been smoking?
Have you ever tried to stop?

Would you like to stop?

Do you use/Have you used . . .

1 cocaine?
2 heroin?
3 other illicit drugs?

How long have you used it?

Have you ever tried to stop?

Would you like to stop?

Have you ever shared needles?
Have you ever shared needles with someone with . . .

1 hepatitis?
2 AIDS?

Do you drink . . .

1 beer?
2 wine?
3 whiskey?

1 cigarrillos?
2 pipa?
3 cigarros?
4 marijuana?

Cuánto fuma al día?

Hace *cuánto* tiempo que fuma?
Ha tratado de *dejar* de fumar?
Le gustaría *dejar* de hacerlo?

Usa/Ha usado . . .

1 cocaína?
2 heroína?
3 otras drogas ilicitas?

Hace cuánto tiempo que la usa?
Ha tratado de dejar de usarla?
Le gustaría dejar de usarla?

Comparte o ha compartido agujas?
Ha compartido agujas con alguien que sufre de . . .

1 hepatitis?
2 SIDA?

Bebe . . .

1 cerveza?
2 vino?
3 whiskey?

4 coffee?	4 ca_fé_?
5 tea?	5 té?

How much each day . . .	Cuánto bebe al día . . .

1 glass?	1 _va_so?
2 bottle?	2 bo_te_lla?
3 cup?	3 _ta_za?

Do you drink when you are . . .	_Bebe_ cuando está . . .

1 alone?	1 _so_lo (a)?
2 sad?	2 _tri_ste?
3 depressed?	3 depri_mi_do (a)?
4 happy?	4 a_le_gre?
5 in a social situation only?	5 en una reunión social sola_men_te?

Do you think you have a drinking problem?	Cree que tiene _problema_ de alcoholismo?
Would you like help?	_Quie_re ayuda?
Do you use any drugs or medicines?	Toma alguna _droga_ o medi_ci_na?
Which ones?	_Cuá_les?
Why do you use them?	_Por qué_ las usa?
How long have you used them?	Hace _cuánto_ tiempo que las usa?
Who gave them to you?	_Quién_ se las dio?

4.4 PAST MEDICAL HISTORY OF THE FAMILY

ANTECEDENTES MÉDICOS FAMILIARES

Is your father (mother) living?	_Vive_ su padre (madre)?
What did he (she) die from?	De qué _murió?_
How old was he (she) when he (she) died?	_Cuántos_ años tenía al morir?

Have you or anyone in your family had . . .[2]		Ha tenido usted o alguién en su familia . . .[2]	
1	high blood pressure?	1	*presión alta?*
2	hyperlipidemia . . .	2	hiperlipidemia . . .
	a high cholesterol?		a *colesterol elevado?*
	b high triglycerides?		b *triglicéridos elevados?*
3	heart disease?	3	enfermedad del corazón?
4	myocardial infarct?	4	*infarto cardíaco?*
5	cerebral infarct?	5	*derrame cerebral?*
6	varicose veins?	6	várices?
7	thrombophlebitis?	7	tromboflebitis?
8	arteriosclerosis?	8	arteriosclerosis?
9	obesity?	9	obesidad?
10	kidney disease?	10	enfermedad de los riñones?
11	diabetes?	11	diabetes?
12	cancer? What type?	12	cáncer? Qué tipo?
13	bronchitis?	13	bronquitis?
14	tuberculosis?	14	tuberculosis?
15	asthma?	15	asma?
16	pneumonia?	16	neumonía?
17	bleeding tendencies?	17	tendencias a *sangrar?*
18	anemias . . .	18	anemias . . .
	a sickle cell?		a células *falciformes?*
	b thalassemia?		b talasemia?
	c iron deficiency?		c *deficiencia de hierro?*
19	convulsions?	19	convulsiones?
20	mental retardation?	20	retraso *mental?*
21	psychiatric problems?	21	problemas *psiquiátricos?*
22	emotional problems?	22	problemas *emocionales?*
23	glaucoma?	23	glaucoma?
24	congenital defects?	24	*defectos de nacimiento*

[2]If the answer is "si," then ask: Quién? (Who?)
Cuándo? (When?)

25 venereal diseases . . .

    a gonorrhea?
    b syphilis?
    c herpes?
    d AIDS?
26 allergies?

Are you allergic to . . .

1 foods . . .
    a eggs?
    b milk?
    c seafood?
2 medicines . . .
    a aspirin?
    b penicillin?
3 pollen?
4 dust?
5 animals . . .
    a dogs?
    b cats?
    c others?

What happens to you?
Have there been any other
diseases?
Which ones?
Is there anything else you
would like to tell me?

25 enfermedades
    venéreas . . .
    a gonorrea?
    b sífilis?
    c herpes?
    d SIDA?
26 alergias?

Tiene *alergia* a . . .

1 las comidas . . .
    a los huevos?
    b la leche?
    c los mariscos?
2 las medicinas . . .
    a la aspirina?
    b la penicilina?
3 el polen?
4 el polvo?
5 los animales . . .
    a los perros?
    b los gatos?
    c otros?

Qué le *pasa*?
Ha padecido de alguna *otra*
enfermedad?
Cuáles?
Hay algo *más* que quiera
decirme?

Chapter 5
CHIEF COMPLAINT OR REVIEW OF SYSTEMS

Chapter 5 begins with a section about pain. In those cases where a detailed analysis of pain and the accompanying circumstances is needed, this section should be consulted. All the organ system sections contain at least the basic questions related to pain. In this way, the interviewer does not always have to refer back to the first section to continue his (her) investigation.

The other questions found in Chapter 6 are necessary for a complete investigation of each organ system. The gastrointestinal system section includes a brief nutritional history. The reproductive system is divided into various subsections: venereal infections, breast examination and pap smear, menstrual history, sexual function, and menopause.

5.1 PAIN

Do you have OR have you had pain?

How long have (did) you had (have) it?

Did it develop . . .

1 slowly?
2 suddenly?

Is this (Was that) the first time that you have (had) this type of pain?
When was the first time?
How long does (did) the pain last each time?
Is (Was) it . . .

1 severe pain?
2 mild?
3 moderate?
4 sharp?
5 intermittent?
6 constant?
7 boring?

EL DOLOR

Tiene O ha tenido dolor?

Cuánto tiempo hace (hacía) que lo tiene (tenía)?

Se *inició* . . .

1 lentamente
2 de repente?

Es (Era) la *primera* vez que le aparece (aparecía)?

Cuándo[1] fue la primera vez?
Cuánto le dura (duraba) cuando le viene (venía)?
Es (Era) un dolor . . .

1 severo?
2 leve?
3 moderado?
4 agudo?
5 intermitente?
6 constante?
7 penetrante?

[1]Whenever using the past tense, ask "cuándo?" (when?). This is important throughout this chapter.

8 colicky?

9 shooting?

10 burning?

11 cramping?

12 pressurelike?

Where is (was) the pain?
Show me with one finger.
Has (Did) the pain changed
(change) location?
Where did the pain begin?
Where does (did) it hurt . . .

1 the most?

2 the least?

Does (Did) the pain radiate?
From where to where?

Do (Did) you have the
pain . . .

1 all the time?

2 in the morning?

3 in the afternoon?

4 at night?

5 before eating?

6 after eating?

7 while eating?

8 when it is (was) cold?

9 when it is (was) hot?

10 when it is (was) humid?

11 when you are (were) . . .
a upset?
b worried?

12 when you exercise
(exercised)?

8 cólico?

9 fulgurante?

10 quemante?

11 como un calambre?

12 opresivo?

Dónde le duele (dolía)?
Señáleme con un dedo.
Ha *cambiado* (cambió) de
lugar?
Dónde le empezó?
Dónde le duele (dolía) . . .

1 más?

2 menos?

Se *corre* (corría) el dolor?
Hacia *dónde?*

Tiene (Tenía) el dolor . . .

1 *todo* el tiempo?

2 por la mañana?

3 por la tarde?

4 por la noche?

5 *antes* de comer?

6 *después* de comer?

7 *mientras* come (comía)?

8 cuando hace (hacía)
frío?

9 cuando hace (hacía)
calor?

10 cuando está (estaba)
húmedo?

11 cuando está (estaba) . . .
a molesto (a)?
b preocupado (a)?

12 cuando hace (hacía)
ejercicio?

13 when you urinate
(urinated) . . .
a at the beginning?
b the whole time?

c at the end?
14 when you defecate
(defecated)?
15 when you have (had)
sexual relations?
16 when you swallow
(swallowed) . . .
a liquids?
b solids?
c both?
17 when you . . .
a stand (stood)?
b sit (sat) down?

c lie (lay) down?

d walk (walked)?
e climb (climbed)
stairs?

f bend (bent) over?

Is (Was) there anything that
makes (made) the pain . . .

1 better?
2 worse?

What is (was) it?
Is (Was) there anything else
that accompanies
(accompanied) the pain?
Does (Did) the pain go away
when you rest (rested)?

13 cuando *orina*
(ori*na*ba) . . .
a al empe*zar*?
b durante *todo* el
tiempo?
c al termi*nar*?
14 cuando *defeca*
·(defe*ca*ba?)
15 cuando tiene (tenía)
*rela*cio*nes sexua*les?
16 cuando *traga*
(tra*ga*ba) . . .
a lí*quidos?
b *só*lidos?
c *ambos?
17 *cuan*do . . .
a está (estaba) *de pie?*
b está (estaba) sen*ta*do
(a)?
c *está (estaba)* acosta-
do (a)?
d ca*mi*na (cami*naba)?
e *su*be *(su*bí*a)*
escaleras?
f se a*ga*cha
(aga*ch*aba)?

Hay (Había) *al*go que . . .

1 lo a*li*vie (alivi*a*ra)?
2 lo au*men*te
(aumen*ta*ra)?·

Qué es (era)?
Hay (Había) otras *mo*les*tias*
que acompañan
(acompañaban) el dolor?
Se a*li*via *(al*ivi*aba)* el dolor al
descansar?

Do (Did) you awake at night from this pain?

Lo *despierta* (despertaba)?

Do (Did) you take anything for the pain?

Toma (Tomaba) algo para el dolor?

Does (Did) it help?

Lo a*livia (aliviaba)?*

Does (Did) it make it worse?

Lo au*menta (aumentaba)?*

Inflammation and Infection

Inflamación e Infección

Do you have OR have you had . . .

Tiene O ha tenido . . .

1 swelling HERE?
2 redness HERE?
3 tenderness HERE?
4 a sensation of warmth HERE?
5 limitation of movement HERE?
6 stiffness HERE?
7 itching HERE?

1 hinchazón AQUÍ?
2 enrojecimiento AQUI?
3 dolor AQUÍ?
4 calor AQUÍ?

5 limitación de movimiento AQUÍ?
6 rigidez AQUÍ?
7 picazón AQUI?

Has pus drained from the wound?

Ha salido *pus* de la herida?

5.2 HEAD AND NECK

CABEZA Y CUELLO

Do you have OR have you had pain HERE?

Tiene O ha tenido dolor AQUI?

What is (was) the pain like?

Cómo es (era) el dolor?

How long have (did) you had (have) it?

Cuánto tiempo hace (hacía) que lo tiene (tenía)?

How long does (did) the pain last each time?

Cuánto le dura (duraba) cuando le viene (venía)?

How often do (did) you have the pain?

Con qué *frecuencia* lo tiene (tenía)?

Does (Did) the pain radiate? From where to where?

Se *corre (corría)* el dolor? *Hacia* dónde?

Is (Was) there anything that makes (made) the pain . . .

Hay (Había) a*lgo* que . . .

1 better?
2 worse?

What is (was) it?

Have you ever been hit in
the . . .

1 head?
2 face?
3 neck?
4 eyes?
5 ears?
6 nose?

Have you ever lost
consciousness?
For how long?
When
What happened?

Do you wear . . .

1 glasses?
2 contact lenses . . .
  a for distance?
  b for close-up?
  c for reading?
  d all the time?
  e since when?

Do you have OR have you
had . . .

  1 frequent . . .
    a headaches?
    b earaches?
    c colds?
    d stuffed-up noses?
  2 many nosebleeds?

1 lo alivie (aliviara)?
2 lo aumente (aumentara)?

Qué es (era)?

Se ha golpeado . . .

1 la cabeza?
2 la cara?
3 el cuello?
4 los ojos?
5 los oídos?
6 la nariz?

Ha perdido el conocimiento?

Por cuánto tiempo?
Cuándo?
Qué le pasó?

Usa . . .

1 anteojos?
2 lentes de contacto . . .
  a para ver de lejos?
  b para ver de cerca?
  c para leer?
  d todo el tiempo?
  e desde cuándo?

Tiene O ha tenido . . .

  1 frecuentemente . . .
    a dolor de cabeza?
    b dolor del oído?
    c catarros?
    d la nariz tapada?
  2 salida de sangre de la
    nariz frecuentemente?

3 many ear infections*?

4 burning of your eyes?
5 itching of your eyes?
6 tearing of your eyes?
7 redness of your eyes?

8 trouble breathing
through your nose?
9 pain . . .
a in your forehead?
b under your eyes?
10 gums that bleed easily?

11 dentures?
12 frequent sores . . .
a on your tongue?
b in your mouth?

When was the last time you
had a . . .

1 vision test?
2 hearing test?

5.3 CARDIOVASCU-LAR-RESPIRATORY SYSTEMS

Do you have OR have you
had . . .

1 pain in your chest?

Where is (was) the pain?
What is (was) the pain like?
How long have (did) you
had (have) it?
How long does (did) the
pain last each time?

3 salida de *pus* de los
oídos (pus coming from
your ears)?

4 *ardor* de los ojos?
5 *picazón* de los ojos?
6 *lagriméo* de los ojos?
7 *enrojecimiento* de los
ojos?

8 *dificultad* al respirar por
la nariz?
9 dol*or* . . .
a en la *frente*?
b *debajo* de los ojos?
10 encías que sangran
facilmente?
11 dentadura *postiza*?
12 úlceras *frecuentes* . . .
a en la *lengua*?
b en la *boca*?

Cuándo fue el *último*
examen especial de . . .

1 la *vista*?
2 los *oídos*?

SISTEMAS CARDIOVASCULAR-RESPIRATORIO

Tiene O ha tenido . . .

1 dolor de *pecho*?

Dónde le duele (dolía)?
Cómo es (era) el dolor?
Cuánto tiempo hace que
lo tiene (tenía)?
Cuánto le dura (duraba)
cuando le viene (venía)?

How often do (did) you have the pain?	Con qué *frecuencia* lo tiene (tenía)?
Is it worse when you breathe?	Es peor cu<u>á</u>ndo respira?
When you inspire/exhale?	C<u>uá</u>ndo inspira/exhala?
Does (Did) the pain radiate?	Se <u>co</u>rre (cor<u>ría</u>) el dolor?
From where to where?	*H<u>a</u>cia* dónde?
Is (Was) there anything which makes (made) the pain . . .	Hay (Había) <u>al</u>go que . . .
a better?	a lo al<u>i</u>vie (alivi<u>a</u>ra)?
b worse?	b lo au<u>me</u>nte (aument<u>a</u>ra)?
What is (was) it?	*Qué* es (era)?

2 shortness of breath . . .
a while exercising?
b at rest?
c when you are (were) upset?
3 difficulty in breathing . . .
a sitting?
b standing?
c lying down?
d exercising?
e at rest?
f when you are (were) upset?
4 night sweats?
5 palpitations?
6 frequent colds . . .
a in winter?
b in spring?
c in summer?
d in fall?

2 sensación de falta de aire?
a al hacer *ejer<u>c</u>icio*?
b al descan<u>sar</u>?
c cuando está (estaba) mo<u>le</u>sto (a)?
3 *dificul<u>tad</u>* para respirar . . .
a sen<u>ta</u>do (a)?
b de pie?
c acos<u>ta</u>do (a)?
d al hacer *ejer<u>c</u>icio*?
e al descansar?
f cuando está (estaba) mo<u>le</u>sto (a)?
4 sud<u>o</u>res por la noche?
5 palpita<u>cio</u>nes?
6 catarros *fre<u>cue</u>ntes* . . .
a en el in<u>vie</u>rno?
b en la prima<u>ve</u>ra?
c en el ver<u>a</u>no?
d en el ot<u>o</u>ño?

7 a cough?
Is (Was) it a dry cough?
Is (Was) it productive?
Is (Was) the phlegm . . .
a foamy?
b thick?
c foul-smelling?
d clear?
e of what color?
f abundant?
g a little bit?
h blood-streaked?

When do (did) you cough?
Do (Did) you have pain
when you cough (coughed)?
Do (Did) you breathe easier
after coughing?

Is (Was) there any position
that makes (made) it . . .

1 better?
2 worse?

Is (Was) the _____
accompanied by . . .[2]

1 fever?
2 chills?
3 sweating?
4 tingling sensation . . .
a in the face?
b in the lips?
c in the extremities?
5 dizziness?
6 nausea?
7 vomiting?

7 tos?
Es (Era) _seca_?
Es (Era) con _flema_?
Es (Era) la _flema_ . . .
a espum_osa_?
b espesa?
c con _mal_ olor?
d _clara_?
e _de qué_ color?
f abun_dante_?
g poco?
h con _manchas_ de
sangre?

A _qué horas_ tose (tosía)?
Le _duele_ (_dolía_) al toser?

Respira (Respiraba) _mejor_
después de toser?

Hay (Había) _alguna_ posición
que . . .

1 la a_livie_ (a_liviara_)?
2 la au_mente_ (au_mentara_)?

Se _acompaña_ (_acompañaba_)
_____ de . . .[2]

1 _fiebre_?
2 escalofríos?
3 su_dores_?
4 hormigueo . . .
a en la _cara_?
b en los _labios_?
c en los _miem_bros?
5 mar_eo_?
6 _náusea_?
7 _vómitos_?

---

[2]Whenever this question form is used, fill in the blank with any of the symptoms found previously.

8 loss of consciousness?

9 fainting?
10 numbness . . .
  a in the lips?
  b in the extremities?
11 pain?

How many pillows do you
sleep with?
Since when?
Have you ever noticed . . .

1 swelling in your . . .
  a feet?
  b hands?
2 bluish color in your . . .
  a lips?
  b feet?
  c hands?
3 coldness in your . . .
  a feet?
  b hands?

What type of regular
exercise do you do?

How many stairs (blocks)
can you climb (walk)
without getting . . .

1 short of breath?
2 pain in your. . .
  a legs?
  b chest?

Does the _____go away
when you stop?

8 *pérdida* del
conocimiento?

9 des*ma*yo?
10 adormeci*mi*ento . . .
  a de los *labios*?
  b de los *miembros*?
11 do*lor*?

con *cuántas* almohadas
duerme?
Desde cuándo?
Ha no*ta*do que . . .

1 se *hin*chan . . .
  a los pies?
  b las manos?
2 se ponen *morados* (as) . . .
  a los *la*bios?
  b los pies?
  c las *ma*nos?
3 se mantienen *fríos* (as) . . .
  a los pies?
  b las *ma*nos?

Qué tipo de *ejercicio* hace
regularmente?

Cuántas escaleras (cuadras)
puede subir (andar) sin
tener . . .

1 una sensación de *ahogo*?
2 do*lor* . . .
  a de las *pier*nas?
  b del cora*zón*?

se *desaparece*_____
cuando para?

5.4 GASTRO-INTESTINAL SYSTEM

SISTEMA GASTROINTESTINAL

Do (Did) you have a good appetite?

Tiene (Tenía) *buen* apetito?

How much do (did) you weigh?

Cuánto pesa (pesaba)?

What is the most/least you've weighed?

Qué fue su peso máximo/mínimo?

Do (Did) you eat . . .

Come (Comía) . . .

1 more than usual?
2 less than usual?
3 the same as usual?

1 *más* que lo usual?
2 *menos* que lo usual?
3 *igual* que siempre?

Are (Were) you on a diet?
Do (Did) you want to gain weight?
Do (Did) you want to maintain your present weight?
Do (Did) you want to lose weight?

Está (Estaba) a <u>dieta</u>?
Quiere (Quería) <u>subir</u> de peso?
Quiere (Quería) <u>mantener</u> su peso actual?
Quiere (Quería) *bajar* de peso?

Has your weight . . .

Su *peso* ha . . .

1 increased?
2 decreased?

1 su<u>b</u>ido?
2 bajado?

How much?
Do you have OR have you had pain in your abdomen?*
Where is (was) the pain?
Show me with one finger.
What is (was) the pain like?
How long have (did) you had (have) it?
How long does (did) the pain last each time?
How often do (did) you have the pain?

Cuánto?
Tiene O ha tenido dolor en el *estómago* (stomach)?
Dónde le duele (dolía)?
Señáleme con un dedo.
Cómo es (era) el dolor?
Cuánto tiempo hace (hacía) que lo tiene (tenía)?
Cuánto le dura (duraba) cuando le viene (venía)?
Con qué *frecuencia* lo tiene (tenía)?

Does (Did) the pain radiate?
From where to where?

Se *corre* (corría) el dolor?
Hacia dónde?

Is (Was) there anything that
makes (made) the pain . . .

Hay (Había) *algo* que . . .

1 better?
2 worse?

1 lo alivie (*aliviara*)?
2 lo aumente (*aumentara*)?

What is (was) it?

Qué es (era)?

Do you get . . .

Le causa . . .

1 indigestion from . . .
2 pain with . . .
 a alcohol?
 b spices?

 c coffee?
 d milk?
 e fats?

1 *indigestión* . . .
2 dol*or* . . .
 a el al*cohol*?
 b la comida
 condiment*ada*?
 c el ca*fé*?
 d la *leche*?
 e las *grasas*?

Do you have OR have you
had problems . . .

Tiene O ha tenido
problemas en . . .

1 swallowing?
2 chewing?

1 tra*gar*?
2 masti*car*?

Do you often . . .

Tiene *frecuentemente* . . .

1 feel nauseated?
2 vomit?
3 burp?

1 *ná*usea?
2 *vó*mitos?
3 er*uc*tos?

When you vomit (vomited),
is (was) it . . .

Cuando *vomita* (*vomitaba*)
es (era) . . .

1 accompanied by
 nausea?
2 before eating?
3 while eating?
4 immediately after
 eating?

1 acompañado de
 náusea?
2 *antes* de comer?
3 *mientras* come?
4 *inmediatamente* después
 de comer?

5 several hours after eating?

6 not related to when you eat (ate)?

7 in large quantities?

8 in small quantities?

9 similar in composition to what you have (had) just eaten?

10 bloody?

11 green?

12 like coffee grounds*?

13 acidic in taste?

14 bitter in taste?

Have you ever noticed . . .

1 black stools?

2 mucus in the stools?

3 bloody stools?

4 fatty stools?

5 foul-smelling stools?

6 foamy stools?

7 clay-colored stools?

8 a yellow color to your skin?

9 itching of your skin?

10 a change in the color of your urine?

11 pain on defecation?

12 anal itching?

13 blood on the toilet paper?

Have you noticed any change in your bowel habits?

How often do you defecate?

When did you last defecate?

---

5 varias horas *después* de comer?

6 *sin relación* con la comida?

7 *mucho?*

8 *poco?*

9 *parecido* a lo que comió?

10 con *sangre?*

11 de color *verde?*

12 de color *café-negro* (color of black coffee)?

13 de sabor *ácido?*

14 de sabor *amargo?*

Ha notado . . .

1 heces *negras?*

2 heces *con moco?*

3 heces con *sangre?*

4 heces con *grasa?*

5 heces con *mal* olor?

6 heces *espumosas?*

7 heces de *color de arcilla?*

8 un color *amarillo* de la piel?

9 *picazón* en la piel?

10 un *cambio* del color de la orina?

11 *dolor* al defecar?

12 *picazón* del ano?

13 *sangre* en el papel higiénico?

Defeca *normalmente?*

Cada cuánto defeca?

Cuándo defecó por la última vez?

Do you have OR have you had . . .

1 constipation?
2 gas?
3 diarrhea?

Since when?
How many times a day do (did) you have diarrhea?
How many times a night?

Is (Was) it accompanied by . . .

1 pain?
2 headache?
3 intestinal cramps?
4 straining?
5 gas?
6 fever?
7 chills?
8 nausea?
9 vomiting?
10 relief after defecating?

Is (Was) the diarrhea . . .

1 of what color?
2 bloody?
3 with fat?
4 with mucus?
5 very foul-smelling?

When you finish (finished), do (did) you feel as if you still have (had) to defecate?

5.4.1 *Nutritional History*

Do you usually eat (drink) . . .

Tiene O ha tenido . . .

1 estreñimiento?
2 gases?
3 diarrea?

Desde *cuándo*?
Cuántas veces al día tiene (tenía) diarrea?
Cuántas veces en la noche?

Se acompaña (acompañaba) de . . .

1 dolor?
2 dolor de *cabeza*?
3 calambres *intestinales*?
4 pujo?
5 gases?
6 fiebre?
7 escalofríos?
8 náusea?
9 vómitos?
10 *alivo* al *terminar* de defecar?

La diarrea es (era) . . .

1 de qué *color*?
2 con *sangre*?
3 con *grasa*?
4 con *moco*?
5 con muy *mal* olor?

Al terminar, se queda (quedaba) con deseos de defecar?

Historia Nutricional

Generalmente come (bebe) . . .

1	bread?		1	pan?
2	rice?		2	ar<u>ro</u>z?
3	beans?		3	frijoles?
4	cereal?		4	cer<u>ea</u>l?
5	macaroni?		5	pastas?
6	green vegetables?		6	vegetales *verdes*?
7	yellow vegetables?		7	vegetales *ama<u>ri</u>llos*?
8	fruits?		8	f<u>ru</u>tas?
9	meats?		9	<u>ca</u>rnes?
10	fish?		10	pes<u>ca</u>do?
11	poultry?		11	<u>a</u>ves?
12	sweets?		12	<u>dul</u>ces?
13	cheeses?		13	quesos?
14	milk?		14	<u>le</u>che?
15	eggs?		15	<u>hue</u>vos?
16	butter?		16	mantequilla?
17	margarine?		17	marga<u>ri</u>na?

Is there anything you don't eat because . . .

Hay *algo* que no come porque . . .

1	you don't like it?		1	no le <u>g</u>usta?
2	it makes you feel bad?		2	le cae *mal*?
3	you are allergic to it?		3	tiene *a<u>le</u>rgia*?
4	it's against your religion?		4	está *en <u>con</u>tra* de su religión?

How many times a day do you eat?
When?
Who prepares the food?

Cuántas veces al día come?

<u>Cuán</u>do?
Quién prepara la comida?

Is the food usually

Es la comida *nor<u>mal</u>mente* . . .

1	raw?		1	<u>cru</u>da?
2	fried?		2	f<u>ri</u>ta?
3	baked?		3	horn<u>ea</u>da?
4	broiled?		4	*a<u>sa</u>da* al fuego?
5	boiled?		5	her<u>vi</u>da?
6	spicy?		6	pi<u>can</u>te?
7	greasy?		7	gra<u>so</u>sa?

8 salty?

How much liquid do you
drink a day?
More or less.
Do you use any sugar
substitute?
Do you take vitamins?
Why?
Which ones?

8 *muy salada?*

Qué cantidad de *líquidos*
toma diariamente?
Más o menos.
Usa algún azúcar *artificial?*

Toma *vitaminas?*
Por qué?
Cuáles?

5.5 URINARY TRACT

Do you have OR have you
had . . .

1 problems with your . . .
   a kidneys?
   b bladder?
2 pain from your . . .
   a kidneys?
   b bladder?

Where is (was) the pain?
What is (was) the pain like?
How long have (did) you
had (have) it?
How long does (did) the
pain last each time?
How often do (did) you
have the pain?
Does (Did) the pain radiate?
From where to where?
Is (Was) there anything
which makes (made) the
pain . . .

   1 better?
   2 worse?

SISTEMA URINARIO

Tiene O ha tenido . . .

1 mol*es*tias de . . .
   a los ri*ñon*es?
   b la ve*ji*ga?
2 do*lor* de . . .
   a los ri*ñon*es?
   b la ve*ji*ga?

Dónde le duele (dolía)?
Cómo es (era) el dolor?
Cuánto tiempo hace (hacía)
que lo tiene (tenía)?
Cuánto le dura (duraba)
cuando le viene (venía)?
Con qué *frecuencia* lo tiene
(tenía)?
Se *corre* (corría) el dolor?
Hacia dónde?
Hay (Había) *algo* que . . .

   1 lo al*iv*ie (aliv*ia*ra)?
   2 lo aumente
      (aument*ara*)?

What is (was) it?	Qué es (era)?
1 pain on urination . . . a at the start? b the whole time? c at the end?	1 dolor al *orinar* . . . a al emp*ezar*? b durante *todo* el tiempo que orina? c al termin*ar*?
2 burning on urination?	2 *ardor* al orinar?
3 to urinate more frequently?	3 que orinar con más *frecuencia*?
4 a feeling of urgency to urinate?	4 *urgencia* para orinar?
5 to urinate in larger quantities?	5 que orinar en *mayores* cantidades?
6 to urinate a lot at night?	6 que orinar *mucho* por la noche?
7 difficulty starting the urinary stream?	7 *dificultad* para empezar a orinar?
8 an interrupted urinary stream?	8 el chorro *interrumpido*?
9 a decrease in . . . a the size of the urinary stream? b the force of the urinary stream?	9 disminu*ción* . . . a del *grueso* del chorro urinario? b de la *fuerza* del chorro urinario?
10 dribbling after urination?	10 *goteo* al terminar de orinar?
11 small stones in your urine?	11 orina con *arenilla*?
12 cloudy urine?	12 orina *turbia*?
13 pink urine?	13 orina *rosada*?
14 urine like Coca-Cola . . . a at the start? b in the middle? c at the end?	14 orina color de *Coca-Cola* . . . a al emp*ezar*? b en el *medio*? c al termin*ar*?

Is (Was) the _____ accom-
panied by . . .[3]

1 fever?
2 chills?
3 malaise?
4 low back pain?

Have you ever involuntarily
dripped urine when you . . .

1 laugh?
2 sneeze?
3 cough?
4 run?

Se acompaña (acompañaba)
_____ con . . .[3]

1 fiebre?
2 escalofríos?
3 malestar general?
4 dolor de la espalda?

Orina por gotas *involuntaria-
mente* cuando . . .

1 se ríe?
2 estomuda?
3 tose?
4 corre?

5.6 REPRODUCTIVE SYSTEM

Do you have OR have you
had pain HERE?
What is (was) the pain like?
How long have (did) you
had (have) it?
When was the last time?
How long does (did) the
pain last each time?
Does (Did) the pain radiate?
From where to where?

Is (Was) there anything
which makes (made) the
pain . . .

1 better?
2 worse?

What is (was) it?

SISTEMA REPRODUCTIVO

Tiene, O ha tenido dolor
AQUI?
Cómo es (era) el dolor?
Cuánto tiempo hace que lo
tiene (tenía)?
Cuándo fue la última vez?
Cuánto dura (duraba)
cuando le viene (venía)?
Se *corre* (corría) el dolor?
Hacia dónde?

Hay (Había) *algo que* . . .

1 lo alivie (aliviara)?
2 lo aumente (aumentara)?

Qué es (era)?

---

[3]Fill in the blank with any of the symptoms found previously.

5.6.1 Venereal Infections

Do you have OR have you
had a genital infection?

With the infection do (did)
you have . . .

1 itching of your genitals?
2 burning of your genitals?
3 redness of your genitals?

4 inguinal swelling?
5 inguinal tenderness?
6 sores on your genitals?
7 pus from the sores?

8 vaginal secretions?
9 fever?

Have you ever had a test
for . . .

1 syphilis
2 gonorrhea
3 herpes
4 AIDS

When?

Were the results . . .

1 positive?
2 negative?

Were you treated?
With what?

5.6.2 Breast Examination and Pap smear

When was your last . . .

1 breast examination?

Infecciones Venéreas

Tiene O ha tenido alguna
infección genital?

Se *acompaña* (*acompañaba*)
la infección con . . .

1 *picazón* de los genitales?
2 *ardor* de los genitales?
3 *enrojecimiento* de los
   genitales?
4 *hinchazón* de la ingle?
5 *dolor* de la ingle?
6 *úlceras* en los genitales?
7 pus *saliendo de las*
   úlceras?
8 *flujo* vaginal?
9 *fiebre*?

Le han hecho una prueba
para . . .

1 sífilis
2 gonorrea
3 herpes
4 SIDA

Cuándo?

Los *resultados* fueron . . .

1 positivos?
2 negativos?

Recibió *tratamiento*?
Con *qué* le trataron?

Examen de los Pechos y Papanicolau

Cuándo fue su *último* . . .

1 examen de los pechos?

2 Pap smear?	2 Papanicolau?
3 mammogram?	3 mamograma?

Were the results . . .

Los *resultados* fueron . . .

1 normal?	1 normales?
2 abnormal?	2 anormales?

Have you noticed . . .

Ha notado . . .

1 a change in the . . .
   a size of your breasts
     (nipples)?
   b shape of your breasts
     (nipples)?
   c consistency of your
     breasts (nipples)?
2 any secretion from the
   nipples?
3 any pain or swelling . . .
   a of your breasts?
   b of your nipples?
   c under your arms?

1 algún *cambio* en . . .
   a el *tamaño* de los
     pechos (los pezones)?
   b la *forma* de los pechos
     (los pezones)?
   c la *consistencia* de los
     pechos (los pezones)?
2 alguna *secreción* de los
   pezones?
3 hinchazón o dolor? . . .
   a de los pechos?
   b de los *pezones*?
   c *debajo* del brazo?

How many children do you
have?
Did you breast-feed them?
Are you breast-feeding now?

Cuántos hijos tiene?
Les dio de *mamar*?
Está dando de mamar
ahora?

Is your . . .

Está circunciso . . .

1 husband circumcised?
2 sexual partner
   circumcised?

1 su esposo?
2 la *persona* con quien
   tiene relaciones sexuales?

5.6.3 *Menstrual History*

Historia Menstrual

How old were you when
your period began?
Do you still have it now?

A *qué edad* le vino su regla
por primera vez?
La tiene *todavía*?

When was your . . .

Cuándo fue su . . .

1   last period?
2   second to last period?

Is your period usually . . .

1   regular?
2   early?
3   late?

How long does it last?

Do you have a . . .

1   light flow?
2   heavy flow?

How many? . . .

1   pads do you use a day?

2   tampons?

How many days pass
between periods?
Do you bleed in between
periods?

With your period do you . . .

1   gain weight?
2   have severe cramps?
3   have breast tenderness?
4   have swelling of your . . .
    a hands?
    b feet?
    c breasts?
5   have back pain?
6   become . . .
    a depressed?
    b emotional?

1   _última_ regla?
2   _penúltima_ regla?

Su regla _normalmente_ es . . .

1   pun_tual_?
2   adelan_tada_?
3   atra_sada_?

Cuánto tiempo le dura?

Sale . . .

1   _poca_ sangre?
2   _mu_cha sangre?

Cuántos (as) . . .

1   toallas sanitarias usa cada
    día?
2   tampónes?

Cada _cuántos_ días le viene?

Sangra _entre_ sus reglas?

Con su _regla_ tiene . . .

1   _aumento_ de peso?
2   cólicos _fuertes_?
3   _dolor_ de los pechos?
4   hincha_zón_ de . . .
    a las _manos_?
    b los pies?
    c los pechos?
5   _dolor_ de espalda?
6   tend_en_cia a . . .
    a depri_mirse_?
    b estar _más_ sensible?

5.6.4 *Sexual Function*

Do you have OR have you
had any change in your
desire to . . .

1 make love with . . .

  a a woman?
  b a man?
2 masturbate?

Do you have OR have you
had any problems with . . .

1 erection? . . .
  a There is (was) none?
  b Is (Was) it difficult to
    achieve?
  c Is (Was) it painful?
2 ejaculation? . . .
  a There is (was none?
  b Is (Was) it difficult to
    achieve?
  c Is (Was) it premature?
  d Is (Was) it painful?
  e Is (Was) it bloody?
3 orgasm? . . .
  a There is (was) none?
  b Is (Was) is difficult to
    achieve?
  c Is (Was) it painful?
4 the quantity of genital
  secretions? . . .
  a Is (Was) it excessive?
  b Is (Was) it too little?

Do you have OR have you
had pain during sexual
relations . . .

1 before intercourse?

Función Sexual

Tiene O ha tenido un
cambio en su deseo de . . .

1 tener *relaciones sexuales*
  con . . .
  a una mujer?
  b un hombre?
2 masturbarse?

Tiene O ha tenido
problemas con . . .

1 la erección? . . .
  a No *la* tiene (tenía)?
  b Le *cuesta* (*costaba*)?

  c Es (Era) *dolorosa*?
2 la eyaculación? . . .
  a *No* hay (había)?
  b Le cuesta (costaba)?

  c Es (Era) prematura?
  d Es (Era) dolorosa?
  e Es (Era) con sangre?
3 el orgasmo? . . .
  a *No* hay (había)?

  b Le cuesta (costaba)?
  c Es (Era) doloroso?
4 la *cantidad de*
  secreciones genitales? . . .
  a Es (Era) excesiva?
  b Es (Era) *poca*?

Tiene O ha tenido dolor
durante sus relaciones
sexuales . . .

1 *antes* del acto sexual?

2 during intercourse?
3 after intercourse?

Are you content with your
sexual relations?
Would you like to talk with a
sexual counselor?

2 *durante* el acto sexual?
3 *despúes* del acto sexual?

Está *satisfecho* (a) con sus
relaciones sexuales?
Quiere hablar con un
consejero sobre el sexo?

5.6.5 Menopause

Have you noticed . . .

1 any change in your
  periods?
2 hot flashes?

3 sweating?
4 dryness of your skin?
5 a decrease in vaginal
  secretions?
6 difficulty or pain with
  entrance of the penis?
7 tiredness?
8 that you are . . .
  a depressed?
  b nervous?
  c irritable?

You are going through
menopause.
This is normal for a woman
of your age.
The symptoms will pass by
themselves.
I can give you something to
make you more comfortable.

La Menopausia

Ha notado . . .

1 algún *cambio* en su
  regla?
2 sensación de *calor* en la
  cara?
3 que suda mucho?
4 *sequedad* de su piel?
5 *disminución* del las
  secreciones vaginales?
6 dificultad o dolor al
  entrar el pene?
7 cansancio? .
8 que *está* . . .
  a deprimida?
  b nerviosa?
  c irritable?

Está pasando por la
menopausia.
Es *normal* para una mujer
de su edad.
Los síntomas pasarán por *sí*
solos.
Peudo darle *algo* para
ayudarle.

5.7 ENDOCRINE SYSTEM

SISTEMA ENDÓCRINO

Do you have OR have you had pain HERE?

Tiene O ha tenido dolor AQUÍ?

What is (was) the pain like?

Cómo es (era) el dolor?

How long have (did) you had (have) it?

Cuánto tiempo hace que lo tiene (tenía)?

How long does (did) the pain last each time?

Cuánto dura (duraba) cuando le viene (venía)?

How often do (did) you have the pain?

Con qué *frecuencia* lo tiene (tenía)?

Does (Did) the pain radiate? From where to where?

Se *corre* (corría) el dolor? *Hacia* dónde?

Is (Was) there anything that makes (made) the pain . . .

Hay (Había) *algo* que . . .

1 better?
2 worse?

1 lo *alivie (aliviara)*?
2 lo *aumente (aumentara)*?

What is (was) it?

Qué es (era)?

Have you OR has anyone else noticed . . .

Ha notado O le han hecho notar . . .

1 a big change in your weight . . .
   a An increase?
   b A decrease?
2 any change in your skin? . . .
   a Is it darker?
   b Is it a finer texture?
   c Is it a rougher texture?
3 any change in your voice? . . .
   a Is it higher?
   b Is it lower?

1 un *cambio grande* en su peso? . . .
   a Ha *subido*?
   b Ha *bajado*?
2 algún *cambio* en su piel? . . .
   a Es *más* oscura?
   b Es *más* fina?
   c Es *más* áspera?
3 algún *cambio* en su voz? . . .
   a Es *más* alta?
   b Es *más* baja?

4 any problem . . .
   a concentrating?
   b sleeping?
5 any change in your breasts? . . .
   a An increase in size?
   b Secretions?

6 any change in the . . .
   a quantity of your total body hair?
   b quantity of hair on your head?
   c color of your hair?
   d texture of your hair?
   e distribution of your hair?
7 any change in your periods?
8 any change in your facial features?
9 any change in your desire for sexual relations?
10 an intolerance to . . .
   a the cold?
   b heat?
11 that you are more tired?
12 that you are more nervous?
13 that you perspire more than usual . . .
   a during the day?
   b at night?
14 that you are more thirsty?
15 that you urinate more?
16 that you eat more?

4 algún *problema* en . . .
   a concen<u>trar</u>se?
   b dor<u>mir</u>?
5 algún <u>cambio</u> en los pechos?
   a Han cre<u>ci</u>do?
   b Han salido secre<u>cio</u>nes?

6 algún <u>cambio</u> en . . .
   a la can<u>ti</u>dad de pelo del cuerpo?
   b la can<u>ti</u>dad de pelo de la cabeza?
   c el <u>color</u> del pelo?
   d la tex<u>tu</u>ra del pelo?
   e la localiza<u>ción</u> del pelo?
7 algún cambio en su <u>regla</u>?
8 algún cambio en su <u>cara</u>?
9 algún cambio en sus de<u>se</u>os sex<u>ua</u>les?
10 que no a<u>guan</u>ta . . .
   a el <u>frío</u>?
   b el ca<u>lor</u>?
11 que se <u>can</u>sa más?
12 que se pone más ner<u>vio</u>so (a)?
13 que suda *más* . . .

   a por el <u>día</u>?
   b por la <u>no</u>che?
14 que tiene *más* sed?

15 que orina *más*?
16 que come *más*?

17 that you eat more and
    do not gain weight?

17 que come *más* y no
    engorda?

When you were a child, did
you ever have radiation
to . . .

De niño (a), recibió *radiación*
en . . .

1 your head?
2 your neck?

1 la ca*be*za?
2 el *cue*llo?

Have you ever noticed a
lump in your neck?

Ha notado una *masa* en el
cuello?

5.8 HEMATOLOGIC SYSTEM

SISTEMA HEMATOLÓGICO

Do you have OR have you
had pain HERE?
What is (was) the pain like?
How long have (did) you
had (have) the pain?
How long does (did) the
pain last each time?
How often do (did) you
have the pain?
Does (Did) the pain radiate?
From where to where?
Is (Was) there anything that
makes (made) the pain . . .

Tiene O ha tenido dolor
AQUÍ?
Cómo es (era) el dolor?
Cuánto tiempo hace que lo
tiene (tenía)?
Cuánto le dura (duraba)
cuando le viene (venía)?
Con qué *frecuencia* lo tiene
(tenía)?
Se *corre* (corría) el dolor?
Hacia dónde?
Hay (Había) *algo* que . . .

1 better?
2 worse?

1 lo *alivie* (aliviara)?
2 lo *aumente (aumentara)*?

What is (was) it?
What is your blood type?
Do (Did) you bruise easily?

Qué es (era)?
Qué tipo de sangre tiene?
Se le hacen (hacían)
moretones sin causa
aparente?

Do (Did) you bleed . . .

Sangra (Sangraba) . . .

1 easily from . . .
   a your nose?
   b your gums?
2 a lot from a cut?
3 for a long time?

1 facilmente de . . .
   a la nariz?
   b las encías?
2 mucho de una herida?
3 por mucho tiempo?

5.9 MUSCULO-SKELETAL SYSTEM

Which hand do you use most . . .

1 the right?
2 the left?
3 both the same?

Do you have OR have you had . . .

1 any broken bones?
2 to wear a brace of any type?
3 muscle weakness?
4 trouble . . .

   a climbing stairs?
   b getting up from a chair?
5 muscle spasms?
6 pain in your . . .
   a bones?
   b muscles?
   c shoulders?
   d elbows?
   e wrists?
   f fingers?
   g hips?
   h knees?
   i ankles?

SISTEMA MÚSCULO-ESQUELÉTICO

Qué mano utiliza más . . .

1 la derecha?
2 la izquierda?
3 igual las dos?

Tiene O ha tenido . . .

1 fracturas?
2 que llevar corsé?

3 debilidad muscular?
4 dificultad en las piernas para . . .
   a subir escaleras?
   b levantarse de una silla?
5 calambres musculares?
6 dolor en . . .
   a los huesos?
   b los músculos?
   c los hombros?
   d los codos?
   e las muñecas?
   f los dedos?
   g las caderas?
   h las rodillas?
   i los tobillos?

Where is (was) the pain?	_Dónde_ le duele (dolía)?
What is (was) the pain like?	_Cómo_ es (era) el dolor?
How long have (did) you had (have) it?	_Cuánto_ tiempo hace que lo tiene (tenía)?
How long does (did) the pain last each time?	_Cuánto_ le dura (duraba) cuando le viene (venía)?
Does (Did) the pain radiate?	Se _corre_ (corría) el dolor?
From where to where?	_Hacia_ dónde?
Is (Was) there anything that makes (made) the pain . . .	Hay (Había) _algo_ que . . .

1 better?	1 lo _alivie_ (_aliviara_)?
2 worse?	2 lo _aumente_ (_aumentara_)?

What is (was) it?	_Qué_ es (era)?

5.10 NERVOUS SYSTEM

SISTEMA NERVIOSO

5.10.1 Cranial Nerves

Nervios Craneales

Do you have OR have you had . . .	Tiene O ha tenido . . .

1 trouble smelling?	1 _dificultad_ para sentir los olores?
2 a sensation of . . . a odd odors? b unpleasant odors?	2 _sensación_ de olores . . . a _raros_? b desagra_dables_?
3 blindness?	3 ce_guera_?
4 blind spots?	4 _manchas negras_ frente a los ojos?
5 blurred vision?	5 vista _nublada_?
6 double vision?	6 visión _doble_?
7 spots before your eyes?	7 _manchas_ enfrente de los ojos?
8 pain behind your eyes?	8 _dolor_ en los ojos?
9 trouble distinguishing colors?	9 _dificultad_ para _distinguir_ los colores?

10	decreased sensation in your face?	10	*pérdida* de la sensibilidad en la cara?
11	trouble chewing?	11	*dificultad* para masticar?
12	Trouble whistling?	12	*dificultad* para silbar?
13	Trouble . . .	13	*dificultad* para . . .
	a opening your eyes?		a *abrir* los ojos?
	b closing your eyes?		b *cerrar* los ojos?
14	decreased taste sensation?	14	*dificultad* para sentir los sabores?
15	taste sensations that are . . .	15	*sensación* de sabores . . .
	a odd?		a *raros*?
	b unpleasant?		b desagra*dables*?
16	loss of hearing?	16	*pérdida* del oído?
17	difficulty in hearing?	17	*dificultad* para oír?
18	the sensation that noises are louder?	18	la *sensación* de que los sonidos son más fuertes?
19	ringing in your ears?	19	*zumbido* en los oídos?
20	trouble swallowing?	20	*dificultad* para tragar?

Since when?[4]

Where?

Did it develop . . .

1 slowly?
2 suddenly?

Has it gotten . . .

1 better?
2 worse?

Desde *cuándo*?[4]

Dónde?

Se ini*ció* . . .

1 lenta*mente*?
2 de re*pente*?

La *molestia* ha . . .

1 mejor*ado*?
2 empeor*ado*?

5.10.2 Sensory

Do you have OR have you had . . .

Sensibilidad

Tiene O ha tenido . . .

---

[4]The following four questions are to investigate any symptoms found in motor and coordination, sensory and cranial nerves.

1 loss of tactile sensation?	1 *falta* de sensibilidad táctil?
2 trouble distinguishing . . .	2 *dificultad* para distinguir . . .
a heat on your skin?	a el *calor* en la piel?
b cold on your skin?	b el *frío* en la piel?
3 tingling sensations?	3 hormigueos?
4 numbness?	4 adormecimiento?

5.10.3 Motor and Coordination

Movilidad y Coordinación

Do you have OR have you had . . .

Tiene O ha tenido . . .

1 loss of coordination?	1 *pérdida* de coordinación?
2 loss of balance?	2 *pérdida* del equilíbrio?
3 dizziness? . . .	3 mareo? . . .
a Did you spin around?	a Daba Vd. *vueltas?*
b Did the objects spin around?	b Le daban *vueltas* los objetos?

5.10.4 Special

Especial

Do you have OR have you had . . .

Tiene O ha tenido . . .

1 loss of . . .	1 *pérdida* del control para . . .
a rectal control?	a defecar?
b bladder control?	b orinar?
2 trouble speaking clearly?	2 *dificultad* para hablar?
3 trouble understanding what you are asked?	3 *dificultad* para entender lo que le preguntan?
4 loss of memory for . . .	4 problemas para *recordar* . . .
a recent events?	a hechos *recientes?*
b past events?	b hechos *pasados?*

5 trouble . . .
  a reading?
  b writing?
6 loss of consciousness?

     5 *problemas* para . . .
      a le*er*?
      b escrib*ir*?
     6 *pérdida* del
       conocimiento?

5.10.5 *Convulsions and Headaches*

Convulsiones y Dolores de Cabeza

Have you ever been hit in the head?

Alguna vez le golpearon la cabeza?

Do you have OR have you had convulsions?

Tiene O ha tenido convul*sion*es?

When did you have your . . .

Cuándo tuvo . . .

1 first convulsion?
2 last convulsion?

1 la *primera* convulsion?
2 la *última* convulsión?

How often do (did) you have them?

Con qué *frecuen*cia le vienen (venían)?

Are (Were) the convulsions preceded by . . .

Están (Estaban) *prece*d*idas* por . . .

1 a special odor?
2 a vision?
3 a constant thought?
4 la strange feeling?
5 any pain?

1 un olor *especial?*
2 una vis*ión?*
3 un pensamiento *fijo?*
4 una sensación *rara?*
5 algún *dolor?*

With the convulsions do (did) you . . .

Con las *convulsiones* . . .

1 lose consciousness?

1 *pierde* (perdía) el conocimiento?
2 se *muerde* (mordía) la lengua?

2 bite your tongue?

How long does (did) each convulsion last?

Cuánto le dura (duraba) cada convulsíon?

After a convulsion, how long are (were) you . . .

1 unconscious?
2 disoriented?

Do (Did) you take medicine for the convulsions?
What kind?
For how long?

Are the convulsions . . .

1 better now?
2 worse now?

Do you have OR have you had headaches?

Are (Were) they . . .

1 mild?
2 moderate?
3 severe?

Where is (was) the pain?
Does (Did) it radiate?
From where to where?
What is (was) the pain like?
How long does (did) the pain last each time?
How often do (did) you have the pain?
In what year did you first have the pain?
When was the last time?

Is (Was) there anything that makes (made) the pain . . .

Después de una convulsión, *cuánto* tiempo . . .

1 está (estaba) *inconciente?*
2 está (estaba) desorient*a*do (a)?

Recibe (Recibía) *tratamiento?*

Qué tipo?
Por *cuánto* tiempo?

Ahora, las convulsiones han . . .

1 mejor*a*do
2 empeor*a*do

Tiene O ha tenido *dolor* de cabeza?

Son (Eran) . . .

1 l*e*ves?
2 moder*a*dos?
3 *fu*ertes?

Dónde le duele (dolía)?
Se *corre* (corría) el dolor?
Hacia dónde?
Cómo es (era) el dolor?
Cuánto le dura (duraba) cuando le viene (venía)?
Con qué *frecuencia* lo tiene (tenía)?
En que año *tu*vo el dolor por primera vez?
Cuándo fue la última *ve*z?

Hay (Habia) *algo* que . . .

1 better?
2 worse?

What is (was) it?

Is (Was) the pain preceded
by . . .

1 a special odor?
2 a vision?
3 a constant thought?
4 a strange feeling?
5 nausea?
6 vomiting?

Is (Was) the pain accom-
panied by other problems?
What?
Are the headaches . . .

1 better now?
2 worse now?

1 lo alivie (*aliviara*)?
2 lo aumente (*aumentara*)?

Qué es (era)?

Está (Estaba) el dolor
precedido por . . .

1 un olor *especial?*
2 una visión?
3 un pensamiento *fijo?*
4 una sensación *rara?*
5 náusea?
6 vómitos?

Siente (Sentía) otras
molestias con el dolor?
Cuáles?
Ahora, los dolores han . . .

1 mejorado?
2 empeorado?

Chapter 6
INSTRUCTIONS FOR THE PHYSICAL EXAMINATION

This chapter begins with the general instructions needed for the physical examination. These particular phrases are repeated only in those organ system sections where they form a large part of the patient's instructions.

As in chapter 5, each organ system has its own section. With the exception of the nervous system, each section contains complete instructions for the physical examination of that particular system. For the examination of cranial nerves II, III, IV, VI, VIII, and IX, the examiner should refer to section 6.2, *Head and Neck*.

The other phrases in this chapter are self-explanatory. However, there are a few points to keep in mind. When the instructions are linguistically complicated, as in the examination of the ocular fundus, the instructions are divided into single phrases. The examiner must remember to employ all the expressions needed to communicate the entire instruction.

Example:

Please . . .	Por favor . . .
1 focus HERE.	1 mire AQUÍ.
2 don't move your eyes.	2 *no* mueva los ojos.
3 don't move your head.	3 *no* mueva la cabeza.
4 don't blink.	4 *no* parpad<u>ee</u>.
5 look into the light.	5 <u>*mire*</u> la luz.

The sections for the urinary tract and the endocrine system are short because of the use of laboratory examinations for diagnosis. There are no instructions for the physical examination of the hematologic system, since this examination is almost exclusively based on observation and laboratory tests.

6.1 GENERAL INSTRUCTIONS

INSTRUCCIONES GENERALES

I am going to examine you. Please undress except for your underwear.

Voy a *examin<u>arle</u>* Por favor desvístese *men<u>o</u>s* su ropa interior.

Please . . .	Por favor . . .
1 lie down.	1 ac<u>ué</u>stese.
2 sit down.	2 si<u>é</u>ntese.
3 stand up.	3 lev<u>á</u>ntese.
4 bend over forward.	4 dóblese hacia *adel<u>a</u>nte*.

5	bend over backward.	5	dóblese hacia *atrás*.	
6	lean forward.	6	inclínese hacia *adelante*.	
7	lean backward.	7	inclínese hacia *atrás*.	
8	lie on your . . .	8	acuéstese . . .	
	a right side.		a sobre el lado *derecho*.	
	b left side.		b sobre el lado *izquierdo*.	
	c stomach.		c boca *abajo*.	
	d back.		d boca *arriba*.	
9	turn your head . . .	9	*mueva* la cabeza . . .	
	a to the right.		a a la *derecha*.	
	b to the left.		b a la *izquierda*.	
10	bend your head.	10	*doble* la cabeza.	
11	turn over.	11	dése *vuelta*.	
12	don't talk.	12	no *hable*.	
13	lie still.	13	quédese *quieto* (a).	

Please do THIS.	Por favor, haga ESTO.
Relax.	Cálmese.
Are you comfortable?	Está *cómodo* (a)?
THIS won't hurt.	ESTO no le dolerá.
Does THIS hurt?	Le duele ESTO?
Can you feel IT?	Puede sentirLO?
I'm sorry if THIS makes you uncomfortable.	Lo siento si ESTO le molesta.
It will only take a moment longer.	Solo un momento *más*.
That's enough.	Suficiente.
Once more.	*Otra* vez.
Very good.	Muy *bien*.
Thank you.	*Gracias*.
You may get dressed now.	Puede vestirse.
I will talk with you when you are finished.	Hablaré con usted cuando *termine*.

6.2 HEAD AND NECK

I am going to examine your . . .

1 head.
2 eyes.
3 ears.
4 nose.
5 mouth.
6 throat.
7 neck.

Do you have pain when I bend your neck?
Please swallow.
Again.

Please . . .

1 read THIS.
2 how many fingers do you see?
3 follow my finger with your eyes.
4 don't move your head.
5 cover your eye like THIS.
6 where do you see my finger?
7 focus HERE.
8 don't move your eyes.
9 don't blink.
10 look into the light.
11 open your eyes.
12 close your eyes.
13 look . . .
   a up.
   b down.
   c to the side.
   d HERE.

EXAMEN FÍSICO DE LA CABEZA Y EL CUELLO

Voy a *examinarle* . . .

1 la cabeza.
2 los ojos.
3 los oídos.
4 la nariz.
5 la boca.
6 la garganta.
7 el cuello.

Tiene *dolor* cuando le doblo el cuello?
Por favor *trague*.
Otra vez.

Por favor . . .

1 lea ESTO.
2 *cuántos* dedos ve?
3 *siga* mi dedo con los ojos.
4 no *mueva* la cabeza.
5 tape el ojo ASÍ.
6 *dónde* ve mi dedo?
7 mire AQUÍ.
8 *no* mueva los ojos.
9 *no* parpadee.
10 *mire* la luz.
11 *abra* los ojos.
12 *cierre* los ojos.
13 *mire* . . .
   a *arriba*.
   b *abajo*.
   c *al lado*.
   d AQUÍ.

I will touch your eye with THIS.	Voy a tocar el ojo con ESTO.
Don't be afraid.	No tenga miedo.

Please tell me . . .

Por favor *digame* . . .

1 when you . . .
   a can hear THIS.
   b cannot hear THIS.
   c can feel THIS.
   d cannot feel THIS.
2 if THIS is . . .
   a louder in one ear.

   b softer in one ear.
   c equal in both ears.

1 cuando . . .
   a pueda oir ESTO.
   b no pueda oir ESTO.
   c pueda sentir ESTO.
   d no pueda sentir ESTO.
2 si ESTO es . . .
   a a *más* fuerte en un oído.
   b *más* suave en un oído.
   c *igual* en ambos oídos.

Breathe through your nose.

Respire por la nariz

Please . . .

Por favor . . .

1 open your mouth wider.
2 stick out your tongue.
3 say "ah."
4 move your tongue from side to side.
5 lift up your tongue.

1 *abra* la boca más.
2 *saque* la lengua.
3 diga "*ah*."
4 mueva la lengua de *lado* a *lado*.
5 *levante* la lengua.

6.3 CARDIOVASCU- LAR-RESPIRATORY SYSTEMS

EXAMEN FÍSICO DE LOS SISTEMAS CARDIOVASCULAR- RESPIRATORIO

I am going to . . .

Voy a . . .

1 examine your lungs.
2 examine your heart.
3 take your pulse.
4 take your blood pressure.

1 examinarle los *pulmones*.
2 examinarle el *corazón*.
3 tomarle el *pulso*.
4 tomar la *presión*.

Please . . .

Por favor . . .

1 sit down.

1 *siéntese*.

2	lean forward.	2	inclínese hacia *adelante*.
3	lie down.	3	acuéstese.
4	lie on your . . .	4	*acuéstese* sobre . . .
	a right side.		a su lado *derecho*.
	b left side.		b su lado *izquierdo*.
5	stand up.	5	levántese.
6	don't talk.	6	*no* hable.
7	breathe deeply through your mouth, . . . again.	7	respire *profundo* con la boca abierta, . . . otra vez.
8	inspire.	8	inspire.
9	hold it.	9	*no* saque el aire.
10	exhale.	10	exhale.
11	take a deep breath.	11	respire *profundo*.
12	relax.	12	descanse.
13	breathe normally.	13	respire *normalmente*.
14	cough.	14	tosa.
15	say "33."	15	diga "*treinta y tres*."
16	say "e."	16	diga "*e*."
17	climb THESE stairs.	17	suba ESTAS escaleras.
18	walk on THIS.	18	camine en ESTO.

Do you feel dizzy?

Se siente *mareado* (a)?

6.4 GASTRO-INTESTINAL SYSTEM

EXAMEN FÍSICO DEL SISTEMA GASTRO-INTESTINAL

I am going to examine your . . .

Voy a examinar su . . .

1	abdomen*.	1	estómago (stomach).
2	rectum.	2	ano.

Please . . .

Por favor . . .

1	try and relax.	1	cálmese.
2	don't cross your legs.	2	*no* cruce las piernas.
3	inflate your stomach.	3	*infle* el estómago.
4	suck in your stomach.	4	*meta* el estómago.

5 take a deep breath.	5 inspire *fuerte*.
6 hold it.	6 *no* saque el aire.
7 relax.	7 descanse.
8 lie on your . . .	8 *acuéstese* sobre su lado . . .
a right side.	a derecho.
b left side.	b izquierdo.
9 bend your leg.	9 *doble* la pierna.
10 straighten out your other leg.	10 *estire* la otra pierna.

6.5 URINARY TRACT

EXAMEN FÍSICO DEL SISTEMA URINARIO

I am going to examine your kidneys.

Voy a examinarle los *riñones*.

Please . . .

Por favor . . .

1 sit up.
2 lean forward.
3 remove your underwear.

1 siéntese.
2 inclínese hacia *adelante*.
3 *quítese* la ropa interior.

Does THIS hurt?

Le duele ESTO.

6.6 REPRODUCTIVE SYSTEM

EXAMEN FÍSICO DEL SISTEMA REPRODUCTIVO

I am going to examine . . .

Le voy a examinar . . .

1 your breasts.
2 your pelvis.
3 your penis.
4 your testicles.
5 for hernias.
6 your genitals

1 los pechos.
2 la pelvis.
3 el pene.
4 los testículos.
5 si tiene *hernias*.
6 los genitales

Do you know how to examine your breasts?
How often do you do it?

Sabe cómo examinarse sus pechos?
Con qué *frecuencia* lo hace?

It is important that you examine your breasts every _____weeks (months). Would you like to learn how?

Es *importante* que Vd. examine los pechos cada _____semanas (meses). Le gustaría *aprender* cómo hacerlo?

Please . . .

Por favor . . .

1 remove your underwear.
2 stand up.
3 cough.
4 bear down.
5 slide closer to the edge of the table.
6 put your legs up HERE.

7 open your legs more.
8 relax your muscles.
9 calm yourself.
10 put your arms like THIS.

1 *quítese* su ropa interior.

2 le*ván*tese.
3 *to*sa.
4 *pu*je.
5 *acér*quese al borde de la mesa.
6 ponga las piernas AQUÍ.
7 *abra* más las piernas.
8 *relaje* los músculos.
9 *cál*mese.
10 ponga los brazos ASÍ.

6.7 ENDOCRINE SYSTEM

EXAMEN FÍSICO DEL SISTEMA ENDÓCRINO

Please swallow
Again.

Trague, por favor.
*O*tra vez.

6.8 MUSCULO-SKELETAL SYSTEM

EXAMEN FÍSICO DEL SISTEMA MÚSCULO-ESQUELÉTICO

Please . . .

Por favor . . .

1 push against my hand as hard as you can.
2 squeeze my fingers as hard as you can.

1 *empuje* fuerte mi mano.

2 *apriete* fuerte mis dedos.

3 don't let me move your . . .
  a head
  b arm
  c leg.
4 raise your . . .
  a arm.
  b leg.
5 relax and let me move your . . .
  a arm.
  b leg.
6 repeat THIS same motion.

3 *no* me deje mover su . . .
  a ca<u>be</u>za.
  b <u>bra</u>zo.
  c <u>pie</u>rna.
4 le<u>van</u>te . . .
  a el <u>bra</u>zo.
  b la pierna.
5 *re<u>lá</u>jese* y déjeme moverle . . .
  a el <u>bra</u>zo.
  b la pierna.
6 repita E<u>S</u>TE mismo movimiento.

6.9 NERVOUS SYSTEM

EXAMEN FÍSICO DEL SISTEMA NERVIOSO

6.9.1 *Mental Status Examination*

Examen del Estado Mental

What is your name?
How old are you?
When were your born?
Where are you?
Why are you here?
Who am I?

Cómo se *lla<u>m</u>a*?
Cuántos años tiene?
En qué *fecha* nació?
Qué lu<u>ga</u>r es *éste*?
Por qué está aquí?
Quién soy?

What . . .

Qué . . .

1 day is this?
2 month is this?
3 year is this?

1 día es *hoy*?
2 mes es *éste*?
3 año es *éste*?

How much is _____ times _____?

Cuánto es _____ por _____?

What did you eat for breakfast?

Qué desayunó?

Who is the President of the United States?

Quién es el presidente de los Estados Unidos?

6.9.2 Cranial Nerves[1]

Nervios Craneales[1]

Does THIS smell like . . .

Huele <u>ESTO</u> a . . .

1 cinnamon?
2 clove?
3 mint?
4 alcohol?
5 tobacco?

1 ca<u>ne</u>la?
2 clavo?
3 <u>men</u>ta?
4 al<u>cohol</u>?
5 ta<u>ba</u>co?

Don't let me open your . . .

No me deje abrir . . .

1 mouth.
2 eyes.

1 Su <u>bo</u>ca.
2 sus <u>o</u>jos.

Please . . .

Por favor . . .

1 smile.
2 whistle.
3 try to close your eyes.
4 shrug your shoulders.
5 don't let me move your head.
6 stick out your tongue.
7 move it from side to side.

1 son<u>rí</u>a.
2 <u>sil</u>be.
3 *intente* cerrar los ojos.
4 le<u>ván</u>te sus hombros.
5 *no* me deje mover su cabeza.
6 <u>sa</u>que la lengua.
7 *mué<u>va</u>la* de lado a lado.

6.9.3 Sensory

Sensibilidad

Close your eyes.
Tell me when you feel SOMETHING.
Where do you feel IT?

<u>Cie</u>rre los ojos.
Dígame cuando sienta <u>AL</u>GO.
Dónde LO siente?

Please tell me if THIS is . . .

Siente <u>ESTO</u> . . .

1 hot.
2 cold.

1 ca<u>lie</u>nte.
2 <u>frí</u>o.

[1]For cranial nerves II, III, IV, VI, VIII, and IX see *Head and Neck* (pp. 64–65).

3 like a prick.
4 like a tap.
5 moving . . .
   a upward.
   b downward.

3 como un *pinchazo*.
4 como un *toquecito*.
5 moviéndose . . .
   a hacia arriba.
   b hacia abajo.

6.9.4 Motor

Please . . .

1 relax.
2 relax your . . .
   a arm.
   b leg.
   c foot.
   d wrist.
3 put your hands like
   THIS.
4 pull as hard as you can.

Movilidad

Por favor . . .

1 cálmese.
2 relaje . . .
   a el brazo.
   b la pierna.
   c el pie.
   d la muñeca.
3 ponga las manos ASÍ.

4 haga *fuerza*.

6.9.5 Coordination

Please . . .

1 close your eyes.
2 keep them shut.
3 stand up with your feet
   together.
4 hold your arms out
   straight.
5 walk heel to toe (LIKE
   THIS).
6 touch my finger with
   your finger and then
   touch your nose.
7 put your heel on your
   ankle.
8 run your heel up and
   down your leg.

Coordinación

Por favor . . .

1 *cierre* los ojos.
2 manténgalos *cerrados*.
3 párese con los pies
   juntos.
4 extienda sus brazos *al
   frente*.
5 camine con un pie
   delante del otro (ASÍ).
6 *toque* mi dedo con su
   dedo y luego toque su
   nariz.
7 *toque* el tobillo con el
   talón.
8 *deslice* el talón sobre su
   pierna.

Do IT faster.
Do IT with the other . . .

1 hand.
2 leg.

HágaLO más rápido.
HágaLO con la otra . . .

1 mano.
2 pierna.

Chapter 7
GENERAL TREATMENT AND FOLLOW-UP

Chapter 7 begins with a section on general therapy. These are patient instructions that do not deal with medications.

Example:
You need to . . .   Necesita . . .

1   stay in bed.   1   *reposar* en cama.
2   avoid excess work.   2   evitar *demasiado* trabajo.
3   take a vacation.   3   tomar vacaciones.

Section 7.2 contains a list of common laboratory examinations. They are grouped in subsections according to organ systems.

In Section 7.3 the technical names of the specialists are given in English. The Spanish translation gives a simplified explanation of each specialty. The literal translation of the Spanish explanation is given in parentheses.

Example:

You need to see . . .

Necesita ver un . . .

1   a cardiologist*.

1   *especialista* en enfermedades de . . .
a el cora<u>zó</u>n (the heart).

7.1   GENERAL THERAPY

TERAPIA GENERAL

You have a problem with your _____.[1]

Tiene un *pro<u>ble</u>ma* con _____.[1]

I don't know what the problem is.

No sé que es *lo que* le molesta.

I want you to see a _____specialist.

Quiero que le *vea* un especialista en enfermedades de _____.

You need to . . .

Necesita . . .

1   have more tests.
2   be hospitalized . . .
a immediately.
b in the near future.
3   stay in bed.
4   relax.
5   sleep . . .
a more.
b less.
6   avoid getting . . .
a upset.
b overtired.
7   get . . .
a more exercise.
b less exercise.

1   *más* pruebas.
2   hospita<u>li</u>zarse . . .
a inmediata<u>men</u>te.
b pró<u>xi</u>mamente.
3   *repo<u>sar</u>* en cama.
4   descan<u>sar</u>.
5   dor<u>mir</u> . . .
a más.
b <u>me</u>nos.
6   evi<u>tar</u> . . .
a moles<u>tar</u>se.
b can<u>sar</u>se.
7   hacer . . .
a *más* ejercicios.
b *<u>me</u>nos* ejercicios.

[1] Throughout this chapter, fill in the blank with the appropriate words.

8   avoid excess work.

9   change jobs to one . . .
    a more active.
    b less active.

10 take a vacation.

11 enjoy yourself more.

12 live in a . . .
    a drier climate.
    b more humid climate.
    c cooler climate.
    d warmer climate.

13 eat . . .
    a more _____.
    b less _____.

14 drink . . .
    a more _____.
    b less _____.

15 never . . .
    a eat _____.
    b drink _____.

16 maintain your weight.

17 try to . . .
    a gain _____pounds.
    b lose _____pounds.
    c stop smoking.
    d stop drinking alcohol.
    e stop using drugs.

18 avoid using your _____.

19 exercise your _____.

20 practice THIS.

21 keep your feet
    elevated . . .
    a all the time.
    b when you rest.

22 avoid straining when
    you defecate.

23 avoid contact with
    _____.

---

8   evitar *demasiado* trabajo.

9   cambiar a un trabajo . . .
    a *más* activo.
    b *menos* activo.

10 tomar *vacaciones*.

11 divertirse *más*.

12 *vivir* en un clima . . .
    a *más* seco.
    b *más* húmedo.
    c *más* frío.
    d *más* caliente.

13 comer . . .
    a más _____.
    b *menos* _____.

14 beber . . .
    a más _____.
    b *menos* _____.

15 no . . .
    a comer _____.
    b beber _____.

16 *mantener* el peso.

17 tratar de . . .
    a *subir* _____libras.
    b *bajar* _____*libras*.
    c *no* fumar más.
    d *no* beber alcohol.
    e no usar drogas.

18 *evitar* el uso de _____.

19 *hacer* ejercicio con
    _____.

20 practicar ESTO.

21 mantener los pies
    elevados . . .
    a *todo* el tiempo.
    b cuando *descansa*.

22 *evitar* esfuerzos cuando
    defeca.

23 *evitar* contacto con
    _____.

24 a cast on your _____.
25 have a transfusion.
26 have an operation . . .
 a immediately.
 b in the near future.

Don't get THIS wet.
You can continue your
sexual activities.
I need your permission to do
THIS procedure.
Please sign THIS permission
sheet.
I want to see you in _____.
Your next appointment
is _____.
Please see the . . .

1 nurse.
2 receptionist.
3 secretary.

24 un yeso en su _____.
25 una transfusión.
26 una operación . . .
 a inmediatamente.
 b próximamente.

No se moje ESTO.
Puede *continuar* sus
actividades sexuales.
Necesito su permiso para
hacer ESTE tratamiento.
Por favor, firme ESTA hoja
de autorización.
Quiero verle en _____.
Su *próxima* cita es
_____.
Por favor, *véase* con la . . .

1 enfermera.
2 recepcionista.
3 secretaria.

7.2 LABORATORY EXAMINATIONS

EXÁMENES DE LABORATORIO

7.2.1 *Head and Neck*

You need a . . .

1
 a vision test.
 b hearing test.
 c test for glaucoma.
2
 a throat culture.
 b nose culture.
 c ear culture.
3 test for allergies.

Cabeza y Cuello

Necesita . . .

1 un examen *especial* . . .
 a de la vista.
 b de los oídos.
 c para glaucoma.
2 un cultivo . . .
 a de la garganta.
 b de la nariz.
 c del oído.
3 una prueba para *alergias*.

4
  a head x-ray.
  b neck x-ray.

7.2.2 Cardiovascular-Respiratory Systems

You need . . .

1 an EKG.
2 an arteriogram.
3 a cardiac catheterization.
4 a chest x-ray.
5 a skull x-ray.

6 a test for . . .
  a cholesterol.
  b triglycerides.
  c exercise tolerance.
  d pulmonary functions.

7 a blood test.
8 bronchoscopy.
9 a lung scan

7.2.3 Gastrointestinal System

You need . . .

1 an upper GI series.

2 a barium enema.
3 a barium swallow.
4 a gastroscopy.
5 a cholecystogram.
6 a colonoscopy.

---

4 una radiografía . . .
  a de la cabeza.
  b del cuello.

Sistemas Cardiovascular-Respiratorio

Necesita . . .

1 un electrocardiograma.
2 un arteriograma.
3 un *cateterismo* cardíaco.
4 una *radiografía* del tórax.
5 una *radiografía* del cráneo.

6 un examen de . . .
  a colesterol.
  b triglicéridos.
  c *tolerancia* al ejercicio.
  d las funciones *pulmonares*.

7 una *prueba* de sangre.
8 una broncoscopía.
9 un centellograma de los pulmones.

Sistema Gastrointestinal

Necesita . . .

1 una *serie* gastrointestinal superior.

2 un enema de *bario*.
3 un trago de *bario*.
4 una gastroscopía.
5 un colecistograma.
6 una colonoscopía.

7 to have . . .
  a a proctoscopic examination
  b a gastric contents analysis.
  c a urine analysis.
  d a stool analysis.
  e a liver function test.
8 a liver biopsy.
9 a stool culture.
10 a liver scan.

11 a blood test.
12 an x-ray of _____.

13 a CAT scan

14 an ultrasound

7 un examen . . .
  a proctoscópico.

  b del *líquido* del estómago.
  c de la orina.
  d de las heces.
  e de la *función* hepática.
8 una *biopsia* del hígado.
9 un *cultivo* de *heces*.
10 un *centellograma* del hígado.

11 una *prueba* de sangre.
12 una radiografía de _____.

13 una tomografía computada

14 un examen de ondas ultrasónicas

7.2.4 Urinary Tract

You need . . .

1 an . . .
  a IVP.
  b retrograde pyelogram.
2 a cystoscopy.
3 to have a . . .
  a urine analysis.
  b renal function test.

  c blood test.
4 a urine culture.
5 a renal biopsy.
6 an x-ray of your _____.

Sistema Urinario

Necesita . . .

1 un pielograma . . .
  a intravenoso.
  b retrógrado.
2 una cistoscopía.
3 un *análisis* de . . .
  a la orina.
  b la función de los riñones.
  c la sangre.
4 un *cultivo* de orina.
5 una biopsia del riñón.
6 una *radiografía de* _____.

7.2.5 Reproductive System

You need . . .

1 to have . . .
  a a breast examination.
  b a pelvic examination.
  c a prostate examination.
  d a blood test.
2 to have . . .
  a a breast biopsy.
  b a uterine biopsy.
  c a prostatic biopsy.
3 a culture . . .
  a of your vaginal secretions.
  b for *Candida*.
  c for *Trichomonas*.
  d for gonorrhea.
  e for syphilis.
  f for herpes.
  g for Chlamydiae.
4 a mammogram.
5 a pap smear.
6 a rectal examination.
7 a semen analysis.
8 a pregnancy test.

9 an x-ray of your _____.

Sistema Reproductivo

Necesita . . .

1 un examen de . . .
  a los pechos.
  b la pelvis.
  c la próstata.
  d la sangre.
2 una biopsia de . . .
  a los pechos.
  b el útero.
  c la próstata.
3 un cultivo . . .
  a de las secreciones *vaginales*.
  b para *Cándida*.
  c para *Tricomonas*.
  d para gonorrea.
  e para sífilis.
  f para herpes.
  g para Chlamydiae
4 una mamografía.
5 un papanicolau.
6 un tacto *rectal*.
7 un análisis del *semen*.
8 una prueba para el embarazo.

9 una radiografía de _____.

7.2.6 Endocrine System

You need . . .

1 an analysis of . . .

Sistema Endócrino

Necesita . . .

1 un *análisis* de la función . . .

a pituitary function.
b thyroid function.
c parathyroid function.
d pancreatic function.
e adrenal function.
f ovarian function.
g testicular function.
2 a glucose tolerance test.

3 an x-ray of your _____.

4 a blood test.
5 a urine analysis.

a de la pituitaria.
b del tiroides.
c del paratiroides.
d del páncreas.
e de los adrenales.
f de los ovarios.
g de los testículos.
2 un examen de *tolerancia* a la glucosa.

3 una radiografía de _____.

4 una *prueba* de sangre.
5 un *análisis* de la orina.

7.2.7 *Hematologic System*

You need . . .

1 a peripheral blood smear.
2 a white cell count.

3 a bone marrow biopsy.

4 to have . . .
a a serum iron analysis.
b a blood clotting test.

c an analysis of your hemoglobin.
d an analysis of your hematocrit.
e an analysis of your blood type.
f a urine analysis.
g a stool analysis.

Sistema Hematológico

Necesita . . .

1 un frote periférico.
2 un *recuento* de glóbulos blancos.

3 una *biopsia* de la médula ósea.

4 un *análisis* . . .
a del *hierro* en la sangre.
b de la *coagulación* de la sangre.
c de la hemoglobina.

d de la hematocrita.

e del *tipo* de sangre.

f de la orina.
g de las heces.

7.2.8 Musculoskeletal System

You need . . .

1 an x-ray of _____.

2 a blood test
3 a urine analysis.
4 to have a . . .
   a bone biopsy.
   b muscle biopsy.
5 a muscle function test.

6 a joint . . .
   a aspiration
   b injection.

Sistema Músculo-Esquelético

Necesita . . .

1 una radiografía
   de _____.

2 una *prueba* de sangre.
3 un *análisis* de la orina.
4 una biopsia de . . .
   a los huesos.
   b los músculos.
5 un examen de la *función muscular*.

6 una . . .
   a *punción* articular.
   b *inyección* intra-articular.

7.2.9 Nervous System

You need . . .

1 an x-ray of your . . .
   a head.
   b neck.
2 an EEG.
3 a brain scan.

4 a cerebral arteriogram.
5 a lumbar puncture.
6 a myelogram.

Sistema Nervioso

Necesita . . .

1 una radiografía . . .
   a de la cabeza.
   b del cuello.
2 un electroencefalograma.
3 un *centellograma* del cerebro.

4 un arteriograma cerebral.
5 una *punción* lumbar.
6 un mielograma.

7.3 SPECIALISTS*

You need to see . . .

1 a specialist in . . .

ESPECIALISTAS*

Necesita ver un . . .

a internal medicine
b otolaryngology

c ophthalmology
d cardiology

e pneumology

f gastroenterology

g nephrology

h gynecology
i endocrinology

j orthopedics

k pediatrics
l hematology
m neurology
n dermatology
o geriatrics
p dental problems
2 a specialist in . . .

a obstetrics

b oncology
c radiology
d psychiatry

e nutrition

1 *especialista* en
enfermedades de . . .?
(specialist in diseases of
. . .)
a los organos internos.
b los oídos, la nariz, la
garganta (ears, nose,
throat).
c los ojos (the eyes).
d el corazón (the heart).
e los pulmones (the
lungs).
f el *aparato digestivo*
(the GI tract).
g los riñones (the
kidneys).
h la mujer (women).
i las hormonas (the
hormones).
j los huesos (the
bones).
k los niños (children).
l la sangre (the blood).
m los nervios (nerves).
n la piel (skin).
o los ancianos (elders).
p los dientes (the teeth).
2 especialista en . . .
(specialist in . . .)
a embarazos y partos
(pregnancy and
delivery).
b cáncer (cancer)
c radiografías (x-rays)
d problemas *emocionales*
(emotional problems).
e *dietas y nutrición* (diet
and nutrition).

3   a psychologist.

4   a surgeon.

3   especialista, no médico, en problemas *emocionales* (nonmedical-doctor, specialist in emotional problems).

4   cirujano.

Chapter 8
MEDICAL THERAPY AND PATIENT INSTRUCTIONS

Chapter 8 is devoted to medical therapy and patient instructions about the use of medications. There are two sections. Section 8.1, Instructions about Medicines, has six subsections that contain the vocabulary needed to explain how medicines should be taken, when they should be taken, and how much should be taken. There are phrases covering previous use of medications, instructions about prescriptions, and a list of possible side effects the patient may experience. The section also contains a series of instructions about the storage of medications.

Section 8.1.6 covers special instructions for the symptoms of insulin overdose and insufficiency. These instructions are written in two forms: the first to communicate directly with the patient and the second to explain the symptoms to family members.

Section 8.2 is an index of some seventy therapeutic and pharmacological classes of medications. It is not a list of medicines by generic or trade name. This information is presented so that the health worker may explain to his patient what type of medicine he or she is taking and why he is taking it.

The different therapeutic and pharmacological groups are listed alphabetically in English by their technical names. The Spanish translation is an explanation of what the medicine is designed to do.

Example:

I am going to treat you with . . .	Le voy a *tratar* con . . .
1 an antiarrhythmic agent.	1 una medicina que *mejora el ritmo de su corazón* (a medicine that improves the rhythm of your heart).

In certain instances, more than just the category of medicine is given. This is done so that the health worker can give more complete information to his patient and still present a simple and understandable explanation.

Example:

I am going to treat you with . . .	Voy a tratarle con . . .
1 insulin that is . . .	1 *insulina de acción* . . .
a short-acting.	a *corta.*
b medium-acting.	b *mediana.*
c long-acting.	c *larga.*

For those health workers who wish to give the specific name of a medication to their patient it is best simply to give the name in English. The patient will probably understand since the names are similar in English and in Spanish. (This is more true for the generic names than for the trade names).

8.1 INSTRUCTIONS ABOUT MEDICINES

INSTRUCCIONES SOBRE LAS MEDICINAS

8.1.1 Prescription Instructions

THIS is a prescription for your medicine.
You can have it filled at any drugstore.
You can renew it
_____ times.
Please call me . . .

1 when you need more.
2 if you do not feel better in _____.
3 if you feel worse.
4 if you have any questions.

Instrucciones Sobre las Recetas

ESTA es una receta para su medicina.
La puede comprar en *cualquier* farmacia.
Puede usar la receta
_____ veces.
Por favor, llámeme . . .

1 cuando necesite *más.*
2 si no se siente *mejor* dentro de _____.
3 si se siente *peor.*
4 si tiene alguna *pregunta.*

8.1.2 Past Use of Medicines

Have you ever taken THIS medicine before?
When?
For what?
How much did you take a day?
For how long?
Did it help?
Did you have any reactions to it?
If you have any reactions, stop the medicine at once and call me.

Empleo Anterior de Medicinas

Ha tomado ESTA medicina antes?
Cuándo?
Para qué?
Qué *cantidad* tomó diariamente?
Por *cuánto* tiempo?
Le *alivió?*
Tuvo alguna *molestia?*

Si tiene *cualquier molestia,* deje de tomar la medicina y llámeme.

8.1.3 How and When to Use the Medicines

I am going to give you an injection.

Take _____

1 pills every _____ hours.

2 teaspoons of syrup every _____ hours.
3 tablespoons of syrup every _____ hours.

Take them for _____

1 days.
2 weeks.
3 months.

Please take the medicine . . .

1 _____ times a day.
2 before meals.
3 with meals.
4 after meals.
5 before bedtime.
6 before you exercise.
7 when you have _____.[1]
8 only when you really need it, because it may be habit-forming.

Drops

Put _____ drops in . . .

1 your nose.

Cómo y Cuándo Usar las Medicinas

Voy a ponerle una *inyección*.

Tome _____

1 píldoras cada _____ horas.

2 *cucharaditas* de jarabe cada _____ horas.
3 *cucharadas* de jarabe cada _____ horas.

Tómelas por _____

1 días.
2 semanas.
3 meses.

Por favor, tome la medicina . . .

1 _____ *veces* al día.
2 *antes* de la comida.
3 *con* la comida.
4 *después* de la comida.
5 *antes* de acostarse.
6 *antes* de hacer ejercicios.
7 cuando tenga _____.[1]
8 *solamente* cuando la necesite mucho porque produce hábito.

Gotas

Ponga _____ gotas en . . .

1 la nariz.

[1]Fill in the blank with the appropriate symptom.

2 your mouth.
3 one eye (both eyes).
4 one ear (both ears).

2 la boca.
3 un ojo (ambos ojos).
4 un oído (ambos oídos).

Cream

Apply the cream to the affected area.

Crema

Aplique la crema en el área afectada.

Spray

Inhale the spray through your . . .

1 nose.
2 mouth.

Spray

Inhale el spray por . . .

1 la nariz.
2 la boca.

Lozenge

Let it dissolve in your mouth.
Let it dissolve under your tongue.
Chew the tablet.

Tableta

Deje que se disuelva en la boca.
Deje que se disuelva debajo de la lengua.
Mastique la tableta.

Powder

Mix_____

1 teaspoons of powder with _____ cups of water.
2 tablespoons of powder with _____ cups of water.

Drink it.
Gargle with the mixture.

Soak your _____ with the mixture for _____ minutes.

Polvo

Mezcle_____

1 cucharaditas de polvo con _____ tazas de agua.
2 cucharadas de polvo con _____ tazas de agua.

Tómela.
Haga gárgaras con la mezcla.

Sumerja su _____ en la mezcla por _____ minutos.

8.1.4 *Common Side Effects*

Efectos Colaterales Comunes

With THIS medicine you may . . .

Con ESTA medicina puede tener . . .

1	be irritable.	1	irritabilidad.
2	be depressed.	2	depresión.
3	be agitated.	3	agitación.
4	have insomnia.	4	insomnia.
5	be dizzy.	5	mareos.
6	feel weak.	6	debilidad.
7	have blurred vision.	7	vista *nublada*.
8	have double vision.	8	visión *doble*.
9	have ringing in your ears.	9	*zumbido* de oídos.
10	note a bad taste in your mouth.	10	un sabor *desagradable* en la boca.
11	have a dry mouth.	11	*sequedad* de la boca.
12	be nauseated.	12	náusea.
13	be thirsty.	13	sed.
14	be hungry.	14	hambre.
15	lose your appetite.	15	*falta* de apetito.
16	have excess salivation.	16	salivación *excesiva*.
17	have diarrhea.	17	diarrea.
18	be constipated.	18	estreñimiento.
19	have a change in the color of your urine.	19	*cambio* de color de la orina.
20	have a different-smelling urine.	20	un olor *especial* de la orina.
21	have more vaginal secretions.	21	*más* flujo vaginal.
22	have palpitations.	22	palpitaciones.
23	have a rash.	23	una erupción.
24	have red spots.	24	*manchas rojas*.

8.1.5 Storage Instructions

Keep THIS medicine . . .

1 at room temperature.

2 in the refrigerator (not in the freezer).
3 out of strong light.

4 in a dry place.
5 away from heat.
6 away from children.

Cómo Guardar las Medicinas

Guarde ESTA medicina . . .

1 a la temperatura ambiente.

2 en el refrigerador (no en el congelador).
3 donde no haya mucha luz.

4 en un lugar seco.
5 fuera del calor.
6 fuera del alcance de los niños.

8.1.6 Instructions for the Diabetic and Family

For the Patient

You should always carry . . .

1 your diabetic ID card.
2 candies.

For Family Members

Help the patient . . .

1 follow his (her) diet.
2 remember to take his (her) insulin.

Instrucciones para el Diabético y la Familia

Para el Paciente

Debe llevar siempre . . .

1 su tarjeta de diabético (a).
2 dulces.

Para los Parientes

Ayude al paciente para que . . .

1 siga su dieta.
2 recuerde usar su insulina.

INSUFFICIENT INSULIN —FOR THE PATIENT

If . . .

1 you do not use enough insulin.

INSUFICIENTE INSULINA —PARA EL PACIENTE

Si . . .

1 no se pone suficiente insulina

2 if you do not follow your diet,

you may . . .

1 · be thirsty.
2 have dry skin.
3 feel nauseated.
4 vomit.
5 faint.
6 have a headache.
7 breathe deeply or rapidly.
8 urinate frequently.

If THIS happens, you must . . . ·

1 ask someone for help.
2 call your doctor.
3 have someone take you to the hospital.

INSUFFICIENT INSULIN —FOR FAMILY MEMBERS

If you notice _____[2]

1 assist the patient with his (her) instructions.
2 call the doctor.
3 take the patient to the hospital.

2 *no come* lo indicado,

puede tener . . .

1 *mucha* sed.
2 piel *seca.*
3 *náusea.*
4 *vómitos.*
5 *desmayo.*
6 *dolor* de cabeza.
7 respiraciones *profundas* o *rápidas.*
8 necesidad de *orinar con más frecuencia.*

Si ESTO le sucede debe . . .

1 *pedir ayuda* a alguien.
2 *llamar* a su *médico.*
3 pedir que *le lleve al hospital.*

INSUFICIENTE INSU- LINA—PARA LOS PARIENTES

Si nota _____[2]

1 *ayude* al paciente con sus instrucciones.
2 *llame al médico.*
3 *lleve al paciente al hospital.*

---

[2] Repeat the symptoms listed under Insufficient Insulin—for the Patient.

INSULIN EXCESS—FOR THE PATIENT

If . . .

1 you use *too much* insulin,
2 you do not follow your diet,
3 you let too much time pass without eating after taking your insulin,
4 you exercise too much,
5 you work too much,

you may . . .

1 feel hungry.
2 be weak.
3 have cold sweats.
4 have blurred vision.
5 be nervous.
6 be dizzy.
7 feel confused.
8 have a headache.
9 faint.
10 have palpitations.

If THIS happens, you must . . .

1 eat or drink something sweet *immediately*.
2 ask someone for help.
3 call your doctor.
4 have someone take you to the hospital.

EXCESO DE INSULINA—PARA EL PACIENTE

Si . . .

1 *se pone demasiada* insulina,
2 *no come* lo indicado,
3 *deja pasar mucho tiempo sin comer* después de ponerse la insulina,
4 hace ejercicio *excesivo*,
5 trabaja *demasiado*,

puede tener . . .

1 hambre.
2 debilidad.
3 sudor *frío*.
4 visión *nublada*.
5 nerviosismo.
6 mareos.
7 confusión.
8 *dolor* de cabeza.
9 desmayos.
10 palpitaciónes.

Si ESTO le sucede, debe . . .

1 comer o beber algo dulce *inmediatamente*.
2 *pedir ayuda* de alguien.
3 *llamar* a su *médico*.
4 *pedir* que le *lleve* al *hospital*.

INSULIN EXCESS— FOR FAMILY MEMBERS

If you notice _____ [3]

1 assist the patient with his instructions.
2 call the doctor.
3 take the patient to the hospital.

If the patient is . . .

1 convulsing
2 unconscious

NEVER give him (her) anything to eat or drink.

8.2 INDEX OF THERA-PEUTIC GROUPS

I am going to treat you with . . .

analgesic that is . . .

1 habit-forming.
2 not habit-forming.

anesthetic that is . . .

1 local.
2 general.

antacid
antialcohol agent

EXCESO DE IN-SULINA— PARA LOS PARIENTES

Si nota _____ [3]

1 *ayude* al paciente con sus instrucciones.
2 *llame a su médico.*
3 *lleve al paciente al hospital.*

Si el paciente está . . .

1 convulsionado(a)
2 inconciente

NUNCA déle nada de comer o beber

INDICE DE GRUPOS TERAPEUTICOS

Le voy a tratar con . . .

una medicina *para el dolor* que . . .
(a medicine for pain that . . .)

1 puede *producir* hábito.
2 no *produce* hábito.

un anestésico . . .

1 local.
2 general.

un antiácido
una medicina que le ayudará a *dejar de tomar alcohol*

[3] Repeat the symptoms listed under Insulin Excess—for the Patient.

	(a medicine that will help you stop drinking alcohol)
antiallergen[4]	una medicina *para las alergias*[4]
antiamebic agent	una medicina *para las amebas*
antianginal agent	una medicina *para el dolor del pecho* (a medicine for chest pain)
antiarrhythmic agent[5]	una medicina *para mejorar el ritmo de su corazón* (a medicine that improves the rhythm of your heart)[5]
antiarthritic agent	una medicina *para el reumatismo*
antibiotic	una medicina *para las infecciones bacterianas*
anticancer agent	una medicina *para el cáncer*
anticoagulant	una medicina que *evita la formación de coágulos*
anticonvulsant	una medicina *para las convulsiones*
antidepressant	una medicina *para la depresión*
antidiarrheal	una medicina *para la diarrea*
antiemetic	una medicina *para los vómitos* (a medicine for vomiting)
antifungal agent	una medicina *para la infección por hongos*
antigout agent	una medicina *para la gota*

[4] If no English translation is given in parentheses, then the Spanish phrase is just an explanation of what the drug does:

antiallergen . . . medicine against allergies.
antidiarrheal . . . medicine against diarrhea

[5] In those cases where the physician does not want to use the specific term, he or she may prefer "una medicina *para su enfermedad* (a medicine for your illness)."

antihelminthic | una medicina *para las lombrices*
(a medicine for worms)

antihemorrhagic agent | una medicina que *evita la hemorragia*

antihistamine | un *antihistamínico*

antihyperlipemic agent | una medicina *para bajar* . . .
(a medicine that lowers . . .)

1 el colesterol
(cholesterol)
2 los triglicéridos
(triglycerides)

antihypertensive agent | una medicina *para bajar su presión*
(a medicine that lowers blood pressure)

anti-flammatory agent | una medicina *para la inflamación*

antimalarial agent | una medicina *para la malaria*

antimanic agent | una medicina *para equilibrar* su estado *emocional*
(a medicine to balance your emotional state)

anti-motion-sickness agent | una medicina *para* . . .
(a medicine for . . .)

1 mareo (dizziness)
2 vértigo (vertigo)

antinauseant | una medicina *para la náusea*

antiparkinson agent | una medicina *para su temblor*
(a medicine for your tremor)

antipsychotic agent | una medicina *para modificar su estado mental*
(a medicine to modify your mental state)

antipyretic agent	una medicina *para bajar la fiebre* (a medicine that lowers fever)
antiseptic	antiséptico
antispasmodic	una medicina *para aliviar los espasmos*
antithyroid agent	una medicina *para bajar la función de la tiroides* (a medicine that lowers thyroid function)
antituberculous agent	una medicina *para tuberculosis*
antitussive agent	una medicina *para la tos* . . . (a cough medicine . . .)
1 with codeine	1 *con codeina*
2 without codeine	2 *sin codeina*
antiviral agent	una medicina *para las infecciones virales*
appetite depressant	una medicina *para quitar el apetito*
appetite stimulant	una medicina *para estimular el apetito*
bronchodilator	una medicina *para respirar más fácilmente* (a medicine that helps you breathe more easily)
decongestant	un descongestionante
digestant	una medicina *para mejorar la digestión* (a medicine that improves digestion)
digitalis	una medicina *para mejorar la función del corazón* (a medicine that improves the function of your heart)

diuretic

una medicina *para orinar más*
(a medicine that makes you urinate more)

emetic

una medicina *para vomitar*
(a medicine that makes you vomit)

fertility agent

una medicina que le *ayudará a tener hijos*
(a medicine that helps you have children)

hematinic

una medicina *para las anemias*
(a medicine that improves anemias)

hematopoietic

una medicina *para producir más sangre*
(a medicine that produces more blood)

insulin that is . . .

insulina de acción . . .

1 short-acting
2 medium-acting
3 long-acting

1 corta
2 mediana
3 larga

laxative

un laxante

muscle relaxant

una medicina que *relaja los músculos*

oral contraceptive

un *anticonceptivo oral*

oral hypoglycemic

una medicina *para la diabetes*
(a medicine for diabetes)

oxytocic

una medicina que *aumenta las contracciones del útero*
(a medicine that increases uterine contractions)

sedative

un sedante

steroids . . .

esteroides . . .

1 androgens

2 corticosteroid that is . . .
   a topical
   b oral
   c injectable
3 estrogens

thyroid drug

tranquilizer
vaccine for _____[6]

vasodilator that is . . .

1 general
2 coronary
3 cerebral

vitamins

1 *hormonas masculinas*
   (male hormones)

2 corticoesteroides . . .
   a tópicos
   b orales
   c inyectables
3 *hormonas femeninas*
   (female hormones)

una medicina *para aumentar
la función del tiroides*
(a medicine that increases
thyroid function)

un tranquilizante
una *vacuna* para _____[6]

una medicina *para mejorar la
circulación* . . .
(a medicine that improves
circulation of . . .)

1 del cuerpo (the body)
2 del corazón
3 del cerebro

vitaminas

_____
[6] Fill in the blank with the appropriate vaccine.

Chapter 9
CONTRACEPTION AND PATIENT INSTRUCTION

This chapter contains five sections. Each one is devoted to instructions for the use of a specific method of contraception. This topic is complicated in any language and, unfortunately, the instructions in Spanish are also long. Whenever possible, the instructions are simplified into a series of phrases. Many of the instructions have been left open-ended so that the health worker may substitute his or her preferred instruction.

Example:

Don't douche for _____ hours after intercourse.[1]	No emplee duchas vaginales hasta después de _____ horas de sus relaciones.[1]
Do you presently use contraception?	Usa *actualmente* anticonceptivos?
Do you use . . .	Usa . . .

[1]Throughout this chapter, fill in the blank with your own specific instructions.

99

1   the pill?
2   the diaphragm?
3   an IUD?

4   foam?
5   vaginal tablets?
6   condoms?
7   the rhythm method?
8   the method of
    withdrawal?
9   abstinence?

Have you had a . . .

1   tubal ligation?
2   vasectomy?

Would you like to have . . .

1   a tubal ligation?
2   a vasectomy?

Are you satisfied with your
present method of
contraception?

1   la *píldora anticonceptiva?*
2   el *diafragma?*
3   el *dispositivo
    intrauterino?*

4   espuma?
5   *tabletas vaginales?*
6   *preservativos* (con*dones*)?
7   el *método del ritmo?*
8   el *método de retirarse
    antes de eyacular?*
9   *abstinencia?*

Le han operado de . . .

1   *ligadura de trompas?*
2   vasectomía?

Le gustaría tener . . .

1   una *ligadura de trompas?*
2   una vasectomía?

Está *satisfecho* (a) con su
método actual?

9.1 INSTRUCTIONS FOR THE BIRTH CONTROL PILL

INSTRUCCIONES PARA LA PILDORA ANTICONCEPTIVA

It is important to follow all
the instructions when taking
the pill.
Take the pill at the same
time each day.

Es importante seguir *todas*
las instrucciones cuando usa
la píldora.
Tome la píldora a la *misma
hora cada día.*

It can be in the . . .

Puede ser por la . . .

1   morning.
2   evening.

1   mañana.
2   noche.

If you forget to take a pill, you must take it before _____ hours have passed. Then take the next pill at the usual hour.

Si *se olvida* tomar una píldora, debe tomarla _antes_ de que pasen _____ horas. Luego, tome la _próxima_ píldora *a la hora* acostumbrada.

With the pill you may . . .

Con la píldora *quizá* . . .

1 gain weight.
2 have . . .
  a enlarged breasts.
  b tender breasts.
3 get headaches.
4 become irritable.
5 have an increased libido.

6 have a decreased libido.

1 *subirá* de peso.
2 tendrá pechos . . .
  a *más* grandes.
  b dolorosos
3 tendrá *dolor de cabeza*.
4 estará *más irritable*.
5 *aumentarán* sus deseos sexuales.
6 *disminuirán* sus deseos sexuales.

There are three types of pills.

Hay *tres clases* de píldoras.

You have the package of . . .

Usted tiene el paquete de . . .

1 21.
2 28.
3 20.

1 veintiuno.
2 veintiocho.
3 veinte.

Package of 21

Paquete de Veintiuno

1 Take the first pill on the fifth day of your period.

1 Tome la *primera píldora* en el *quinto día* de su regla.

2 Day 1 of your period is the first day you bleed.

2 El *primer día* de su regla es el *primer día* que sangra.

3 Take the pills daily for 3 weeks.

3 Tome las píldoras diariamente *durante tres semanas*.

4 Then stop for 7 days.

5 Your period will come on the second or third day after you finish the package.

6 Begin the next package on the same day of the week that you finished the other pack.

7 If your period does not start, begin the next pack as indicated.

Package of 28

1 Take the first pill on the fifth day of your period.

2 Take THESE for 3 weeks.

3 Take THESE daily for the next 7 days.

4 On the eighth day begin a new pack.

5 Your period will begin on the second or third day after you begin the last row of pills (THESE taken for 7 days).

6 You must take a pill every day.

7 If your period does not start, begin the next pack as indicated.

4 Luego para *durante siete días*.

5 Su regla vendrá el *segundo o tercer día* después de terminar el paquete.

6 Empiece el próximo paquete *el mismo día* de la semana en que terminó el otro paquete.

7 Si su regla no viene, *continúe* con el próximo paquete como está señalado.

Paquete de Veintiocho

1 Tome la *primera píldora* en el *quinto día* de su regla.

2 Tome ÉSTAS durante tres semanas.

3 Tome ÉSTAS diariamente durante los próximos siete días.

4 Al *octavo día* empiece un nuevo paquete.

5 Su regla vendrá el *segundo o tercer día después de empezar* la *última fila* de píldoras (*LAS* que tome durante los siete días).

6 Hay que tomar una píldora *cada día*.

7 Si su regla no viene, *continúe* con el próximo paquete como está señalado.

Package of 20

1   Take the first pill on the fifth day of your period.

2   Take a pill daily for 20 days.

3   Then stop for 6 days.

4   Your period will come on the second or third day after you stop taking the pills.

5   Begin the new pack on the same day of the week that you finished the other pack.

6   If your period does not start, begin the next pack as indicated.

Paquete de Veinte

1   Tome la *primera píldora* en el *quinto día* de su regla.

2   Tome una píldora diariamente durante *veinte días*.

3   Luego para durante seis *días*.

4   Su regla vendrá el *segundo o tercer día después de terminar* las píldoras.

5   *Empiece* el nuevo paquete *el mismo día* de la semana en que *terminó* el otro paquete.

6   Si su regla no viene, *continúe* con el próximo paquete como está señalado.

9.2 INSTRUCTIONS FOR THE DIAPHRAGM

You can put it in place _____ hours before having intercourse.
Don't forget to put the special cream on the diaphragm before putting it in.
You can remove the diaphragm _____ hours after intercourse.

INSTRUCCIONES PARA EL DIAFRAGMA

Puede ponerlo _____ *hora(s) antes* de tener relaciones sexuales.
No se olvide de poner la crema especial en el diafragma *antes* de ponérselo.
Puede *quitarlo* _____ *horas después* de las relaciones.

9.3 INSTRUCTIONS FOR THE CONDOM, FOAM, AND VAGINAL TABLET

INSTRUCCIONES PARA EL PRESERVATIVO, LA ESPUMA Y LA TABLETA VAGINAL

When used alone . . .

Cuando se usa _solo_ (a) . . .

1 the condom is not very safe.

2 foam is not very safe.

3 the vaginal tablet is not very safe.

1 el preservativo, (el condón), _no es muy seguro_

2 la espuma _no es muy segura_

3 la tableta vaginal _no es muy segura_

But it is better than nothing at all.

Pero es _mejor_ que usar nada.

It is better to use . . .

Es _mejor_ usar . . .

1 foam with a condom.

2 vaginal tablet with a condom.

1 la espuma _con un preservativo (un condón.)_

2 la tableta vaginal _con un preservativo (un condón.)_

Insert the . . .

Póngase . . .

1 foam _____ hour(s) before intercourse.

2 vaginal tablet _____ hour(s) before intercourse.

1 la espuma _____ _hora_(s) _antes_ del acto sexual.

2 la tableta vaginal _____ _hora_(s) _antes_ del acto sexual.

The man should wear the condom whenever he enters the vagina, not only during intercourse.

El hombre _debe_ usar el preservativo _cada vez_ que el pene tiene contacto con la vagina, _no sólo durante_ el verdadero acto sexual.

Don't douche for _____ hours after intercourse.

No emplee duchas vaginales _hasta después de_ _____ _ho_ras de sus relaciones.

It inactivates the effects of the foam and vaginal tablet.

Inactiva los efectos de la espuma y de la tableta vaginal.

9.4 INSTRUCTIONS FOR THE IUD

INSTRUCCIONES PARA EL DISPOSITIVO INTRAUTERINO

Would you like to use an IUD?
I can fit one for you.
When the IUD is in its proper place, the string will always be the same length.
You can check the length by inserting your finger.
Try IT now.

Le gustaría usar el *dispositivo intrauterino*?
Puedo *colocarle* uno.
Cuando está bien colocado *debe tocar* el *hilo siempre a la misma distancia*.
Puede *comprobarlo* introduciendo el dedo.
HágaLO ahora.

9.5 INSTRUCTIONS FOR THE RHYTHM METHOD

INSTRUCCIONES PARA EL MÉTODO DE RITMO

This method is most advisable for a woman who has very regular periods.
You can have intercourse _____ days before your period begins and _____ days after the last day of your period.
You should not have intercourse any other time unless you can use another type of contraception.

Este método es aconsejable a las mujeres que tienen su *regla puntualmente*.
Puede tener relaciones sexuales _____ días *antes de que* comience la regla y _____ días *después del* último *día* de la regla.
No se debe tener relaciones los demás días, a *menos que* se emplee *otro método* de anticoncepción.

Chapter 10
PREGNANCY AND DELIVERY

The three sections of this chapter cover history of past pregnancies and deliveries, present pregnancy, and present delivery. The questions and instructions are self-explanatory.

10.1 HISTORY OF PAST PREGNANCIES AND DELIVERIES

How many times have you been pregnant?
How many children do you have?
Did you breast-feed them?

Have you ever had . . .

  1 babies that were . . .
     a large?
     b small?

HISTORIA DE PARTOS Y EMBARAZOS ANTERIORES

Cuántas veces ha estado embarazada?
Cuántos hijos tiene?

Les dió de *mamar*?

Ha tenido . . .

  1 niños . . .
     a grandes?
     b pequeños?

c premature?
d congenitally
  malformed?
2 multiple births . . .

a twins?
b more than two?
3 a forceps delivery?
4 a cesarean?
5 a child that was
  born . . .
  a feet first?
  b with the cord around
    the neck?
6 a child that was born
  dead?
7 a child that died shortly
  after birth?

8 problems with the
  placenta?
9 a postpartum hemor-
  rhage?
10 a miscarriage?
11 an abortion?

How many weeks pregnant
were you when you had . . .

1 the abortion?
2 the miscarriage?

How long was your labor
with the . . .

1 first child?
2 other children?

How much did your children
weigh?

c prematuros?
d con *defectos* de
  nacimiento?
2 nacimientos
  múltiples . . .
  a gemelos (as)?
  b *más* de dos?
3 un parto con *forceps*?
4 una cesárea?
5 un niño que haya
  nacido . . .
  a *de pies*?
  b con el cordón
    alrededor del cuello?
6 un niño que haya
  nacido *muerto*?
7 un niño que haya
  muerto poco después
  de nacer?
8 algún *problema* con la
  placenta?
9 una *hemorragia después*
  del parto?
10 un aborto *espontáneo*?
11 un aborto *provocado*?

Cuántas semanas de
embarazo tenía cuando tuvo
el aborto . . .

1 provocado?
2 espontáneo?

Cuánto le duró el trabajo de
parto con . . .

1 su *primer* niño?
2 sus *otros* niños?

Cuánto pesaron sus niños?

10.2 PRESENT PREGNANCY

EMBARAZO ACTUAL

I am going to examine you.
What is the date of your last period?

Le voy a *examinar*.
Cuándo fue su *última* regla?

Do you have OR have you had . . .

Tiene O ha tenido . . .

1	anxiety?	1	ansie*dad*?
2	depression?	2	depre*sión*?
3	irritability?	3	irritabili*dad*?
4	sleepiness?	4	s*ueño*?
5	insomnia?	5	ins*omn*io?
6	headaches?	6	*dolores* de cabeza?
7	vision problems?	7	molestias de la *vista*?
8	convulsions?	8	convul*sion*es?
9	nausea?	9	*ná*usea?
10	vomiting?	10	v*ómi*tos?
11	constipation?	11	estreñimiento?
12	loss of appetite?	12	*pérdida* de apetito?
13	craving for special foods?	13	antojos?
14	urinary problems?	14	molestias *urinarias*?
15	a lot of vaginal secretions?	15	*mucho* flujo vaginal?
16	tiredness?	16	cans*ancio*?
17	low back pain?	17	do*lor* de la espalda?
18	swelling of your feet?	18	*hinchazón* en los pies?
19	varicose veins?	19	*vári*ces?
20	hemorrhoids?	20	hemo*rro*ides?
21	difficulty in breathing?	21	*dificultad* para respirar?
22	high blood pressure?	22	*presión alta*?

You are _____ weeks pregnant.
Was this a planned pregnancy?

Usted tiene _____ semanas de embarazo.
Estaba *planeado* este embarazo?

Do you want to . . .

Quiere . . .

1 continue with the pregnancy?
2 have an abortion?

Do you want to breast-feed this child?
Do you have any hereditary diseases?

10.3 PRESENT DELIVERY

How close together are the pains?
How long do they last?

Do you know if . . .

1 a lot of water has come out?
2 blood has come out?

I am going to examine you.
You are _____ centimeters dilated.
Do you need to urinate?

I am going to . . .

1 shave you.
2 clean you.
3 give you an enema.

You will have to . . .

1 wait patiently.
2 tell me when you have a pain.
3 slide closer to the edge of the table.
4 put your legs up HERE.
5 relax your muscles.

1 *seguir* con el embarazo?
2 tener un aborto *provocado*?

Quiere darle de *mamar* a este niño?
Tiene alguna enfermedad *hereditaria*?

PARTO ACTUAL

Cada cuánto le vienen los dolores?
Cuánto le duran?

Sabe si . . .

1 ha salido *mucha* agua?
2 ha salido *sangre*?

Le voy a *examinar*.
Tiene _____ centímetros *de cuello*.
Tiene deseos de *orinar*?

Voy a . . .

1 rasurarle.
2 limpiarle.
3 darle un *enema*.

Tendrá que . . .

1 esperar *tranquilamente*.
2 avisarme cuando tenga un *dolor*.
3 acercarse *al borde* de la mesa.
4 poner las piernas AQUÍ.
5 *relajar* sus músculos.

6 calm yourself.
7 breathe slowly through your mouth.
8 pant.
9 push only when you are told.
10 conserve your strength.
11 rest between pains.

12 have an episiotomy.
13 have stitches.

It is a . . .

1 boy.
2 girl.

He (she) weighs
_____ pounds and
_____ ounces.
He (she) is healthy.
Would like to see your baby?

6 calmarse.
7 respirar *lentamente* por la boca.
8 jadear.
9 empujar solo cuando le diga.
10 *conservar* su fuerza.
11 *descansar* cuando no tenga dolor.

12 tener una *episiotomía*.
13 tener *puntos*.

Es . . .

1 un niño.
2 una niña.

Pesa _____ *libras* y
_____ onzas.

Es sano (a).
Le gustaría *ver* a su niño (a)?

Chapter 11
POISONING
AND PATIENT
INSTRUCTION

This final chapter is designed to aid the health worker in cases of intoxication. It contains a list of the more common poisonous agents, immediate instructions for the patient or other party to follow, and a list of general symptoms associated with the various intoxicants.

The text is written in two styles. The first is a set of instructions directed to a third party. For example, a parent calls or brings the child to the hospital because she suspects he (she) has swallowed a poison. The second style is the same set of instructions directed to the patient him- or herself.

The chapter ends with general instructions designed to explain how to help avoid future problems of this nature.

11.1 COMMON INTOXICANTS

What did he (she, you) swallow?
[I don't know.][1]
[I think it is . . .

1 a medicine . . .
  a aspirin.
  b amphetamines.
  c barbiturates.
  d tranquilizers.
  e antiallergen.
  f cough syrup.
  g contraceptives.
  h antiseptics.
2 alcohol.
3 a cleaning agent . . .
  a Clorox.
  b furniture polish.
  c a disinfectant.
  d a detergent.
4 an insecticide.
5 a hair dye.
6 lead from . . .
  a paint.
  b metal toys.
  c batteries.
7 a plant.
8 a mushroom.
9 spoiled food . . .
  a milk and milk products.
  b canned goods.]

INTOXICANTES COMUNES

Qué tomó?

[No sé.][1]
[Creo que *es* . . .

1 una medi_ci_na . . .
  a aspi_ri_na.
  b anfeta_mi_nas.
  c barbit_ú_ricos.
  d tranquili_zan_tes.
  e antial_ér_genicos.
  f ja_ra_be para la tos.
    anticoncep_ti_vos.
  h antis_é_pticos.
2 alco_hol_.
3 un líquido *limpia_dor_* . . .
  a _clo_ro.
  b una *cera para muebles*.
  c un des_in_fec_tan_te.
  d un deter_gen_te.
4 un insecti_ci_da.
5 un *tinte para el pelo*.
6 _plo_mo de . . .
  a pin_tu_ra.
  b *juguetes* de metal.
  c bate_rí_as.
7 una _plan_ta.
8 un _hon_go.
9 una comida *pa_sa_da* . . .
  a *_le_che y deri_va_dos*.

  b productos *enla_ta_dos*.]

---

[1]The square brackets indicate possible responses to the patient or third party.

When did he (she, you) swallow it?	*Cuándo* lo tragó?
How much did he (she, you) swallow?	*Cuánto* tragó?
Call THIS number _____.	Llame a ESTE número _____.

11.2 INSTRUCTIONS DIRECTED TO A THIRD PARTY

Do the following . . .

1 give him (her) . . .
  a milk.
  b egg whites.
  c vinegar.
  d strong tea.
  e black coffee.
  f mineral oil.
  g antacid.
2 induce vomiting with . . .
  a your finger.
  b mustard and water.
  c salt and water.
3 bring him (her) to the hospital immediately.

11.3 INSTRUCTIONS DIRECTED TO THE PATIENT

Do the following . . .

1 drink . . .
  a milk.
  b egg whites.
  c vinegar.

INSTRUCCIONES DIRIGIDAS A OTRA PERSONA

Haga lo siguiente . . .

1 *déle* . . .
  a *leche*.
  b *clara* de huevos.
  c *vinagre*.
  d té *fuerte*.
  e café *negro*.
  f aceite *mineral*.
  g *antiácido*.
2 hágale *vomitar* con . . .
  a su *dedo*.
  b agua con *mostaza*.
  c agua con *sal*.
3 tráigale al hospital *inmediatamente*.

INSTRUCCIONES DIRIGIDAS AL PACIENTE

Haga lo siguiente . . .

1 tome . . .
  a *leche*.
  b *clara* de huevos.
  c *vinagre*.

d strong tea.
e black coffee.
f mineral oil.
g antacid.

2 induce vomiting with . . .
a your finger.
b mustard and water.
c salt and water.
3 come to the hospital
immediately.

d té *fuerte*.
e café <u>negro</u>.
f aceite mine<u>ral</u>.
g antiá<u>c</u>ido.

2 *vomite* con . . .
a su <u>de</u>do.
b agua con *mos<u>ta</u>za*.
c agua *con sal*.
3 venga al hospital
inmedia<u>tamen</u>te.

11.4 COMMON SYMPTOMS

SÍNTOMAS COMUNES

Does he (Do you) have OR
has he (have you) had . . .

Tiene O Ha tenido . . .

1 dizziness?
2 irritability?
3 sleepiness?
4 insomnia?
5 depression?
6 excitability?
7 convulsions?
8 paralysis?
9 confusion?
10 incoordination?

11 constipation?
12 nausea?
13 vomiting?
14 diarrhea?
15 abdominal pain?
16 headache?
17 respiratory difficulty?
18 palpitations?
19 blue fingers?
20 blue lips?

1 ma<u>re</u>o?
2 irritabili<u>dad</u>?
3 *mucho* sueño?
4 ins<u>om</u>nia?
5 depre<u>sión</u>?
6 excita<u>ción</u>?
7 convul<u>siones</u>?
8 pa<u>rá</u>lisis?
9 confusión *men<u>tal</u>*?
10 pérdida de
coordinación?
11 estreñimiento?
12 <u>náu</u>sea?
13 <u>vó</u>mitos?
14 dia<u>rre</u>a?
15 <u>có</u>licos abdominales?
16 *do<u>lor</u>* de cabeza?
17 dificultad *respira<u>to</u>ria*?
18 palpita<u>ciones</u>?
19 dedos *mo<u>ra</u>dos*?
20 labios *mo<u>ra</u>dos*?

21	small pupils?	21	pupilas *pequeñas*?
22	large pupils?	22	pupilas *grandes*?
23	blurred vision.	23	vista *nublada*?
24	a dry mouth?	24	*sequedad* de la boca?

11.5 INSTRUCTIONS FOR PREVENTION OF FUTURE INTOXICATIONS

ALWAYS keep all medicines and poisons . . .

1 away from children.

2 in a locked cabinet.

3 in a high place.
4 in their original containers.
5 labeled clearly.

NEVER keep medicines and poisons . . .

1 with food.
2 in food containers such as . . .
   a milk bottles.
   b pop bottles.

INSTRUCCIONES PARA LA PREVENCIÓN DE INTOXICACIONES FUTURAS

SIEMPRE guarde medicinas y substancias peligrosas . . .

1 donde los niños *no las alcancen*.

2 en un gabinete cerrado con *llave*.

3 en un sitio *alto*.
4 en su caja *original*.

5 con una etiqueta clara.

NUNCA guarde medicinas y substancias peligrosas . . .

1 donde hay *comida*.
2 en un *recipiente* para la comida como . . .
   a botellas de *leche*.
   b botellas de *soda*.

Chapter 12
AIDS AND PATIENT INSTRUCTION

12.1 INFORMATION FOR THE PATIENT

AIDS is an infection caused by a virus.

SIDA es una infeccion causada por un virus.

The virus is called HIV.

El virus se llama HIV.

HIV is transmitted by blood products and sexual relations.

HIV se transmite por productos de sangre y relaciones sexuales.

HIV weakens the body's defenses to infection.

HIV debelita las defensas del cuerpo contra infeccion.

It can take years of infection with HIV before one develops AIDS.

Puede estar infectado con HIV por años antes de tener SIDA.

There is a blood test to detect whether you have been infected by the AIDS virus.

Hay un examen de sangre para detectar si usted esta infectado por el virus que causa AIDS.

The blood test is not perfect, but it is extremely accurate.

El examen de sangre no es perfecto, pero es muy exacto.

I need your permission to perform this blood test.

Necesíto su permiso para hacer este examen de sangre.

The results of the blood test will be kept confidential.

El resultado del examen sera confidencial.

Although there is no cure for AIDS at this time, there are many helpful treatments.

Aun que ahora no hay un curato para SIDA, hay muchos tratamientos effectivos.

Patients with AIDS sometimes get infected with viruses, bacteria, or funguses.

Pacientes con SIDA algunas veces sufren de infecciones de viruses, bacteria, o hongos.

PCP, or pneumocystis, is a type of lung infection that many AIDS patients get.

PCP, o pneumocystis, es una infeccion del pulmon del cual sufren muchos pacientes con SIDA.

There is inhaled and intravenous medicine for PCP.

Hay medicina inhalada y intravenosa para PCP.

Kaposi's sarcoma is a tumor that some AIDS patients get.

La sarcoma de Kaposi es un tumor del cual sufren algunos pacientes con SIDA.

The lesions of Kaposi's sarcoma can affect the skin, intestines, lungs, or brain.

Las lesiones de la sarcoma de Kaposi se encuentran en la piel, los intestinos, los pulmones, o el cerebro.

There are medical treatments, including chemotherapy, for Kaposi's sarcoma.

Hay tratamientos, incluyendo chemoterapia contra la sarcoma de Kaposi.

You must be careful not to infect your mate with the HIV virus.

Tiene que ser prudente para no infectar su companero(a) con el virus de HIV.

You must use a condom when having intercourse.

Tiene que usar un condon cuando tiene coito.

Friends and family members with whom you are not intimate are not at risk of getting AIDS from you.

Amigos y miembros de la familia con los cuales usted no tiene relaciones intimas, no tienen peligro de contractar SIDA de usted.

Appendix
GENERAL
VOCABULARY

A.1   DAYS, MONTHS, HOLIDAYS

Days of the Week[1]	Días de la Semana[1]
Monday	lunes
Tuesday	martes
Wednesday	miércoles
Thursday	jueves
Friday	viernes
Saturday	sábado
Sunday	domingo

Months of the Year	Meses del Año
January	enero
February	febrero
March	marzo
April	abril
May	mayo
June	junio
July	julio
August	agosto
September	septiembre
October	octubre
November	noviembre
December	diciembre
today	hoy
yesterday	ayer
tomorrow	mañana

[1]In Spanish, days of the week and months of the year are not capitalized.

day before yesterday	anteayer
day after tomorrow	pasado mañana
last year	el año pasado
last month	el mes pasado
last week	la semana pasada
this year	este año
this month	este mes
this week	esta semana
next year	el año próximo
next month	el mes próximo
next week	la semana próxima

Holidays

Días de Fiesta

Christmas	Navidad
New Year	Año Nuevo
Valentine's Day	Día del cariño
Easter	Pascuas
Holy Week	Semana Santa
July 4	Cuatro de julio
Halloween	Día de todos los Santos
birthday	cumpleaños
anniversary	aniversario

A.2 CARDINAL AND ORDINAL NUMBERS

NÚMEROS CARDINALES Y ORDINALES

Cardinal Numbers

1	uno	14	catorce
2	dos	15	quince
3	tres	20	veinte
4	cuatro	30	treinta
5	cinco	40	cuarenta
6	seis	50	cincuenta
7	siete	60	sesenta
8	ocho	70	setenta
9	nueve	80	ochenta
10	diez	90	noventa
11	once	100	cien

12	doce	1000	mil
13	trece	1,000,000	millón

Other numbers are made by adding two numbers

10 + 6	diez y seis
10 + 7	diez y siete
20 + 1	veinte y uno or veintiuno

Ordinal Numbers

first	primero (a)	seventh	séptimo (a)
second	segundo (a)	eighth	octavo (a)
third	tercero (a)	ninth	noveno (a)
fourth	cuarto (a)	tenth	décimo (a)
fifth	quinto (a)	eleventh	décimo primero (a)
sixth	sexto (a)	twelfth	décimo segundo (a)

A.3 TIME EXPRESSIONS

EXPRESIONES DEL TIEMPO

hour	hora
minute	minuto
second	segundo
at noon	al medio día
at midnight	a la media noche
in the morning[2,3]	por la mañana[2], durante la mañana[3]
in the afternoon	por la tarde, durante la tarde
in the evening	por la noche, durante la noche

The word "time" has three translations

1 What TIME is it?   Qué HORA es?

In this instance "time" is translated as "hora" (hour).

---

[2] When "in" is translated as "por," the expression refers to "morning" as a short interval of time, no specific hour.
[3] When "in" is translated as "durante," the expression refers to "morning" as a larger interval of time, but still no specific hour.

2   Take the medicine three
    TIMES a day

Tome la medicina tres
VECES al día.

Here the word "time" refers to time in a series. It is used for a repeated action. ("Vez" is the singular form of "veces".)

3   I have TIME to see you
    today.

Tengo TIEMPO para verle
hoy.

"Tiempo" is used to express time in the sense of duration.

What time is it?

Qué hora es?

Between the hour and the half hour, *add* the number of minutes to the hour.

Example:
It is 3:00 in the afternoon.[4]
It is 3:10. (It is 3 AND 10.)
It is 3:30.[5]
It is 3:15.[6]

Son las tres de la *tarde*.[4]
Son las tres Y diez.
Son las tres y *media*.[5]
Son las tres y *cuarto*.[6]

Between the half hour and the next hour, *subtract* the number of minutes from the next hour.

Example:
It is 3:40. (It is 4 MINUS 20.)

Son las cuatro MENOS
veinte.

It is 3:45.
It is 3:55.

Son las cuatro menos cuarto.
Son las cuatro menos cinco.

The third-person plural form of the verb "ser" (to be) is "son." When telling time, this form is used with every hour except 1 o'clock, for which the singular form "*es*" is used.

Example:
It is 1:00.
It is 1:20.

Es la una.
Es la una y veinte.

[4] When a specific hour is given,

in the morning		de la mañana
in the afternoon	are translated as	de la tarde
in the evening		de la noche

[5] *media:* one-half, 30 minutes
[6] *cuarto:* one-quarter, 15 minutes

It is 1:30.
It is 12:50.

Es la una y media.
Es la una menos diez.

A.4 COLORS

What color is it?
red
white
green
blue
black
brown
gray
yellow
purple
pink

COLORES

De qué color es?
rojo (a)
blanco (a)
verde
azul
negro (a)
café
gris
amarillo (a)
morado (a)
rosado (a)

A.5 CONTRASTING ADJECTIVES

large
small

tall (for height)
short (for height)

high
low

long (for length)
short (for length)

fat
thin

heavy (for weight)
light (for weight)

dark (for colors)
light (for colors)

ADJETIVOS QUE CONTRASTAN

grande
pequeño (a)

alto (a)
bajo (a)

alto (a)
bajo (a)

largo (a)
corto (a)

gordo (a)
flaco (a), delgado (a),
seco (a)

pesado (a)
liviano (a), ligero (a)

oscuro (a)
claro (a)

round	redondo (a)
square	cuadrado (a)
rectangular	rectangular
triangular	triangular
oval	ovalado (a)
smooth	liso (a)
rough	áspero (a), rugoso (a)
regular	regular
irregular	irregular
curly	rizado (a), crespo (a)
straight	liso (a)
soft	suave
hard	duro (a)
tepid	tibio (a)
hot	caliente
boiling	hirviendo
wet	mojado (a)
dry	seco (a)
humid	húmedo (a)
open	abierto (a)
closed	cerrado (a)
painful	doloroso (a)
painless	sin dolor
many	muchos (as)
some	algunos (as)
few	pocos (as)
mobile	móvil
immobile	inmóvil
flat	plano (a)
raised	elevado (a)
central	central
peripheral	periférico (a)

loud	fuerte
soft	suave
weak	débil
strong	fuerte
symmetric	simétrico (a)
asymmetric	asimétrico (a)
better	mejor
worse	peor
the best	lo mejor
the worst	lo peor
alive	vivo (a)
dead	muerto (a)
healthy	sano (a)
sick	enfermo (a)
sweet	dulce
sour	agrio (a)
bitter	amargo (a)

A.6 WEIGHTS AND MEASURES

PESOS Y MEDIDAS

length	longitud
width	ancho
height	altura
volume	volumen
weight	peso
gram	gramo
kilogram	kilogramo
liter	litro
square millimeter	milímetro cuadrado
square centimeter	centímetro cuadrado
cubic centimeter	centímetro cúbico
millimeter	milímetro
centimeter	centímetro

milligram	mili̲gramo
microgram	micro̲gramo

A.7 PHRASES FOR THE FIRST VISIT

EXPRESIONES PARA LA PRIMERA VISITA

Come in please.	*Entre*, por favor.
My name is _____.	Me llamo _____.
Who is the patient?	*Quién* es el paciente?
What is your name?	Cómo *se llama*?
It's nice to meet you.	Mucho *gusto* en conocerle.
Did you come alone?	Vino *solo* (a)?
Who brought you?	*Quién* le trajo?
I would like to talk with you now.	*Me gustaría* hablar con usted ahora.
Later I will examine you.	*Más tarde* le voy a examinar.

INDEX OF TERMS

Terms used in this index without page numbers do not appear in the text. They are included with the Spanish translation for reference purposes only. An Index of Verbs follows this index.

INDEX OF VERBS

135

ISBN 0-07-006489-X

90000>

9 780070 064898